ULTIMATE
HEALTH

LIVE LONGER · BE LEAN · BE STRONG!

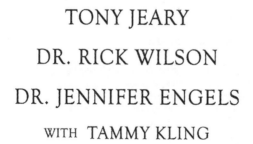

TONY JEARY

DR. RICK WILSON

DR. JENNIFER ENGELS

WITH TAMMY KLING

Carpenter's Son Publishing

Ultimate Health: Live Longer*Be Lean*Be Strong!

© 2013 by Tony Jeary, Rick Wilson, Jennifer Engels, Tammy Kling

Published by Carpenter's Son Publishing, Franklin, Tennessee

Cover Design by Debbie Manning Sheppard

Interior Layout Design by Suzanne Lawing

Written / Edit by Tammy Kling

Printed in the United States of America

978-0-9885931-0-7

Table of Contents

Section II - Reference Lists of 25

Section III - Health Tools

Some strive for wealth, yet ignore the health required to enjoy it.
Consider your mortality and invest in healthy habits.

—Dr. Rick Wilson

INTRODUCTION

Why did you pick up this book?

Chances are it is because the title appeals to you.

Ultimate Health is seductive, because we all want it. We all want to live longer, healthier, more energetic lives. But how many of us take an active role in actually creating it?

If you're like many people, you plan for your career, family, and financial future. You consider the vacation and health benefits that go along with a job before accepting it. You analyze the location and resale value of a home before purchasing it so that your investment is protected. You plan ahead for your family, setting aside money for your kids' college education. Most people plan for their future—but what about your health?

Remarkably, many people neglect their greatest asset, leaving their health to chance. They live life on autopilot, focused on achieving their goals and daily activities without thinking of the consequences of every daily habit and choice. But it's these daily choices that matter, and that's why I assembled this team to write this book.

As an author and corporate strategist, I've been blessed to work with some of the most brilliant CEO minds on earth. I've helped entrepreneurs, athletes, and high achievers all across the globe reach even higher levels of success, and at times a common thread has been the pursuit of achievement—and neglect of overall health.

Pursuing business goals can put people on a treadmill that takes them away from maintaining a focus on physical health. But, our physical lives and business lives are integrated, and if you're stressed emotionally or not feeling well physically, it affects the way you perform at work. When I coach business leaders today, we often end up discussing the health of their business, their cultures, their families, and their own individual lives.

My 50th year on this earth has been the best year of my life so far. One of the best things that happened was a positive report from my extensive physical exam at the renowned Cooper Clinic in Dallas, TX. I dropped 25 pounds and increased my energy and vitality that year! I have lived this book. I have lost 40 pounds and I'm down to 11% body fat. I've shaved 6.5

inches from my waist and I feel healthier than ever. I am proud to say that I have truly reached another level. But what does "another level" *really* mean as it pertains to our health?

You can live in ultimate health if you make the decision to—today. Each one of us has been uniquely created, yet there are specific preventive things we can do individually to strengthen our bodies, minds, and health to live longer and stronger.

We can take preventive measures to eliminate stress, resist the onset of disease, and turn back the clock. The majority of diseases can be prevented by lifestyle changes and early detection. But you can't change what you don't know, so this book is a guide to create awareness.

One of the most common illnesses, for instance, is cardiovascular disease. And most people don't know that cardiovascular disease can be preventable by changes in lifestyle. When you stop unhealthy habits such as smoking or living a sedentary life, and adopt healthy ones such as exercise and eating your greens, you increase your cardiovascular health. Brain incidents such as stroke, which is the fourth-leading killer in the United States, can be prevented by changes in diet and lifestyle as well. Understanding critical factors like your hormone levels, platelet and white cell count, blood sugar, and vitamin and nutrient levels, are all important to maintaining ultimate health—and all are within reach via a simple blood test. The focus of this book is on guiding you toward the prevention that can save lives!

> But you can't change what you don't know, so this book
> is a guide to create awareness.

The Johari Window concept suggests we should examine not only what we know, but also what we don't know that we don't know. Instead of "ignorance is bliss," I believe we should seek to understand the truth. Knowledge really is power when it comes to your health. We want to shatter the old paradigm of "sick care." Today, prevention matters. We want to show you how to take your own health into your hands.

Almost every month we hear about some celebrity who died unnecessarily because they have invested everything in their careers, and every other aspect of their lives, yet haven't had screenings, whole body CT scans, treadmill stress testing, or other preventive exams. Then all is suddenly lost with the unexpected fatal event. Cancer is discovered too late to achieve a successful life-saving intervention. Disease processes have gone unchecked for too long. Today, a quality life can be lengthened with simple lifestyle modifications and basic preventive tests; we have the tools and the technology!

Optimal health is the integration of preventive medical elements to achieve the best results-oriented outcomes. Instead of simply relying on a default approach that turns to pharmaceuticals or surgery first, the better strategy is to take a preventive approach. My friend and coauthor, Dr. Wilson, on staff at the world renowned Cooper Clinic in Dallas, Texas, is also my doctor. As a dermatologist, he saves lives and has trained a staff of professionals who know what to look for in screenings for cancerous growths and other critical conditions. Dr. Wilson also looks ten years younger than his 66 years and even leg presses 450 pounds! I'd say he's an example of Ultimate Health. He is also passionate about illuminating our need for wellness instead of sick care.

As I started learning more about health and preventive medicine from my research and my team of doctors, it became readily apparent that I had been living with multiple blind spots concerning my health management. I started a dialogue with Dr. Wilson about his research, and we developed an intriguing presentation that I began sharing with my executive clients. The reaction was powerful—much stronger than I expected!

We put together a powerful team to write this book, and it includes Jennifer Engels, MD, who served as a preventive radiologist at the Cooper Clinic and is an expert in nutrition; international Best-selling author and life wellness coach Tammy Kling; and Matt Engels, MD, an anesthesiologist. In addition, we have consulted with a number of wellness experts and physicians around the globe to write a book that would impact thinking and save lives.

The United States Census Bureau predicts more than half a million centenarians (people who live to be 100) by the year 2050. Yet you have probably believed the traditional assumption that your lifespan would last to only somewhere in your seventies. But what if you could extend your life and live an even richer, fitter, more peaceful, more energetic lifestyle each day—starting today? What if you could boost your immune system and strengthen your brain to live vibrantly like Jack Lalane, or like Helen Small, a Dallas woman who—in her 90s!—wrote a book, got her MBA, and got a new job with a prestigious teaching hospital?

We wrote this book to change your beliefs about aging and longevity. We want to guide you to developing helpful habits that will add years to your life and life to your years!

In the following chapters, we are going to challenge your beliefs about what health really is, and ignite you to gain total clarity about what you want and how healthy you want to become. We have selected twenty areas that can have the most impact on your health, and we've developed a personal assessment for you as a starting point.

In the Ultimate Health Assessment, take a look at each of the twenty areas and rate yourself from 1-5, with 5 being the highest. How well do you manage stress? How often do you exercise? Are you getting the required amount of sleep to sustain brainpower? This assessment is the first step toward discovering the areas in which you need to improve or modify in order to live in ultimate health.

As a CEO coach and strategist, part of my work involves helping high achievers reach their maximum potential. CEOs are busy by nature and, although they are disciplined, it is not uncommon for them to work so much that they neglect their health.

In these pages, I'd like to encourage you to not only survive but to thrive, learn, and grow. Let me be your coach, and join me and the rest of my expert medical team as we embark on a journey to transform each day into an abundant life full of healthy choices and outcomes.

Ultimate Health is a surgical intervention against unbalanced life priorities which prevent us from functioning at our healthy best. It fills our knowledge gaps providing clarity of principles and motivation for healthy longevity.

—**Kenneth E. Salyer, MD**, World renowned craniofacial surgeon / crusader for children who suffer from head and facial deformities.

Ultimate health is a practical preventive medicine reference and healthy longevity tool. It reflects my personal experience that exercise and movement play a pivotal role for experiencing quality of life with longevity.

—**Orville C. Rogers**, holder of six USA Track and Field world indoor running records from 60 meters to 3000 meters for age group 95 to 99.

As an elite athlete in football and powerlifting and then Naval Special Operations Officer, I was blessed with the best performance advisors, trainers, and fitness minds in the US. Transitioning into my third and best career as husband, father and steward of God's gift of my life, I now fully realize how great a blessing it is to have access to the insight, encouragement, and wisdom of excellent coaches.

The authors of Ultimate Health have now stepped into that role providing a practical, actionable guide for an extended quality life.

—**Clint Bruce**, retired Navy SEAL, founder of Carry the Load and Trident Response Group

Total life prosperity is the path to ultimate health and it's a concept that 1 percenters understand. It's about being healthy (not balanced) in all quadrants. Mind, body, and soul. Faith, family, fitness and finances.

—**Tammy Kling**, Author, *Freedom, Live and Dream*

I exercise for at least an hour a day. I also take classes at a nearby college. I exercise my body and my brain!

—**Jim Potticary**, 85 years young

ULTIMATE HEALTH
ASSESSMENT

Rate yourself on a scale of 1 to 5, with 5 being the highest,
on your current effectiveness in each area.

#	Category	Description	Rating
1.	Lifestyle	How are you living your life? Managing balance, managing risks, resting, saying "no" enough, and exercise all make up your overall living routine. Are your habits supporting your health?	
2.	Mental Management	What goes on in our minds truly impacts our health. Assess your own self-talk, your daily attitude, and your beliefs about being healthy and not getting sick; your willingness to release grudges and forgive, while focusing on the positives. Filter the input you receive from sources such as news, media, or even negative people.	
3.	Ultimate Longevity	Do you have a great team of health professionals that know you and guide you? Family doctor? Nutritionist? Dentist? Do you have regular checkups and vaccines? Do your behaviors align with real health?	
4.	Stress Management	Are you managing anxiety? Are you meditating? Relaxing enough? Is your life aligned with your values? Have you set up harmony in your life so things run as smoothly as possible? Is your pace of life contributing to or detracting from your overall well-being?	
5.	Immune System	Your immune system protects you. It detects potential harm and helps your body react. Are you helping yourself? Are you resting at the right time, for example, when you sense your body needs it to ensure you stay well? Are you maintaining good hygiene; protecting against harmful bacteria; practicing plain and simple cleanliness such as washing your hands enough and avoiding being in contact with the wrong things in order to support your wellness?	
6.	Testing	Early detection is great common sense in today's world of information. How is your discipline on staying current on screenings, blood work reviews, EKGs, MRIs, hormones testing, and urinalysis—even full-body skin screenings every few years? There are many simple things we can do to be proactive. Are you taking advantage of these options?	

7.	Exercise	Physical exercise matters—regular, frequent, and ongoing. Resistance exercise, cardiovascular exercise (aerobics), balance, and stretching all promote a better-operating body.	
8.	Oral	Obviously, it is important to keep your mouth clean. Are you brushing enough? Flossing enough? Going for regular check-ups?	
9.	Eyes/ Vision	Are you protecting your eyes from sunlight and eating the things that help prevent cataracts later in life? Are you going for regular checkups? Do you wear eye protection when doing certain types of work around the house? All these factors add up to promoting this key component to your body's overall health.	
10.	Toxin Management	What's around you can get in your body through your skin, what you breathe, and what you eat. Toxins are potentially hazardous substances that can place an extra toll on your body such as forcing your liver and kidneys to work overtime as they filter fluids. Are you protecting yourself like you could or should?	
11.	Hormone Management	A hormone is a chemical released by a cell or a gland in one part of your body that sends out messages that affect cells in other parts of your body. In essence, it's a chemical messenger that transports a signal from one cell to another. Have you tested your chemical balances (estrogen, testosterone, thyroid, DHEA, etc.)? Are you supplementing where you should?	
12.	Vitamins	A vitamin is an organic compound required as a vital nutrient in tiny amounts by an organism. Vitamins help your body function optimally. Are you managing your regular intake, testing so you know, and living daily with the right balances in your body?	
13.	Caloric Management	A calorie is a unit of energy. It is a measure of the energy we generate with every task we do, as well as a measure of the energy delivered by a food we eat. How well do you know your body and how you balance what you eat versus what you need to perform? Being in tune and knowing this can allow you to make better daily choices . . . and live better!	
14.	Ear, Nose, and Throat	Preventive testing is important for the ear, nose, and throat, the same as for the rest of your body. It is important to protect your hearing and ear canal from foreign objects and loud noises. Are you maintaining good hygiene? Are you getting checked regularly?	
15.	Food	Food is any substance consumed to provide nutritional support for your body. It is usually of plant or animal origin, and contains essential nutrients, such as carbohydrates, fats, proteins, vitamins, and minerals. It is what we consume in an effort to produce energy, maintain life, and stimulate growth. How is your balance? How is your mix? Are you eating throughout the day to promote good metabolism? Do you eat slowly and chew well in order to promote good digestion? Do you make healthy choices such as limiting the fried, processed, and high-sugar foods you eat?	

16.	Skin	Your skin is the largest organ in your body. It acts as an external filter and can even provide many clues about the condition of your body internally. Are you protecting it like you should from ultraviolet rays or from harmful chemicals that can get into your body? Do you get full-body skin screenings to detect cancers or other harmful things that need attention in order to ensure your ultimate health? Skin cancer is the most common cancer there is.	
17.	Fluids	Consuming adequate amounts of water is critical to maintaining ultimate health. Do you drink enough water each day? Do you manage your alcohol intake? Do you drink too much soda or other high-sugar drinks?	
18.	Emotions	Emotion is a complex psycho-physiological experience of your state of mind as you interact with internal and external influences. How are your mood, temperament, personality, disposition, and motivation? All these elements matter; all impact the way our bodies perform.	
19.	Sleep	Sleep suspends the sensory activity of nearly all voluntary muscles. It accentuates the growth and rejuvenation of the immune, nervous, skeletal, and muscular systems. Are you getting enough sleep? Is it good sleep?	
20.	Spiritual well-ness	Your spiritual wellness is to a large degree reflective of your worldview. Is it egocentric or others oriented? Would others say you display stress tolerance and adequate marginal reserves for life's challenges? What wisdom do you apply to your life situations in order to achieve spiritual balance, peace and joy?	

Your Total: _____

INTERPRETING YOUR TOTAL

A 100 is exceptional—and exceptionally rare. This is not designed to be a scientific assessment, but an awareness tool.

> **5-20: Red flag**
> **21-55: Average**
> **56-80: Above average**
> **80-100: Excellent**

Take action in the areas in which you need to improve.

Take charge of your health and, in the following chapters, learn about the steps you can take to live a healthier and more energetic life.

Section I

This book is a living tool. It's designed with you and your daily life in mind. It's a kitchen counter book—not a coffee table book.

Keep it on the kitchen counter, and flip through it during the day as a constant reminder of your goal of living in ultimate health. When you reach for something in the refrigerator, prepare a meal, or entertain a guest at the counter, your health manual for life will be at your fingertips. This book is intentionally basic and designed for simplicity. Each chapter offers simple yet life-saving tools for living, some of which you may have heard before, but overlooked. We have collaborated on this book for you, to remind you that it's never too late to live younger, stronger, and longer.

CHAPTER 1
LIFESTYLE

How are you living your life? Are you balanced or unbalanced? Do you feel stressed or at peace? Do you manage risks, get enough rest, and say no when you need to? All of these lifestyle factors combined, along with nutrition and regular exercise, contribute to a positive outcome. Are your daily habits supporting a healthy life?

How you live your life each day determines how long and how healthy it will be. Your longevity and youth are in your hands, not in your DNA, as most people believe. Your youthful look, skin, muscle tone, and internal organ function is primarily the result of the choices you make each and every day. A fit, healthy, and nutrient- and exercise-rich lifestyle leads to an outcome of abundant energy, vitality, and youth! This is the truth, and we hope to help you live it by making you more aware of the things you can do to lengthen and strengthen your life.

Successful people are self-aware. The questions and statements at the beginning of every chapter are designed to help you recalibrate and understand where you are—in order to know where you need to be.

How healthy are you?

Not just physically, but also emotionally, spiritually, mentally, and in all quadrants of your life. *Ultimate Health* means having complete clarity about the life you want and taking the preventive and proactive measures required in order to live it.

What does being the best, the strongest, and the healthiest mean to you? Does it mean achieving a lower cholesterol level, exercising three times a week, or incorporating more antioxidants into your diet? Or maybe you have set a goal to spend more time with yourself, perhaps writing or meditating on your goals. The two are more closely related than you think. You need a balanced mental and physical approach to your health to truly be at your best.

Throughout this book you will see the term "ultimate health" many times: not just health—*ultimate* health. We all joined together to write this book because we share the same passion: to live in Ultimate Health and educate others about how they can transform their lives and do the same.

Ultimate Health means having complete clarity about the life you want and taking the preventive and proactive measures required in order to live it.

LIVING TEN YEARS YOUNGER

Sometimes all it takes to look and feel younger is changing one or two habits in your life. Chances are you know someone who has lost twenty pounds or more and transformed their body. If you have ever witnessed that, you've seen how a reduction in excess body fat can make someone look younger! The same goes for people who smoke. Smoking can make the skin appear dry, wrinkled, and much older than it actually is. Eliminating one bad habit can turn back time.

And here's why it's important.

No one knows how long they're going to live. Any of us could live to be 80, or for decades more. But the key to long life isn't just existing, it is living a quality life! A life where you can be active and have a passion, curiosity, desire to learn, and joy about your life until your last day.

The United States government predicts that by the year 2050 there will be over half a million centenarians. Hard to imagine! Nearly half a million people living to 100! That means that if you are 70, you could live to be one 100. It is possible. The question becomes, then, what kind of life will it be? Are you doing what you can to thrive and increase your longevity?

Many people suffer with diseases that could have been prevented by simply living a better life! Diseases like obesity, diabetes, heart disease, high blood pressure, and depression. (Yes, even depression!) Thinking about your daily habits and decisions now can prevent deficiencies in lifestyle later.

No matter where you live, what you do for a living, or who you are, your health is up to you. You are responsible for your body and how healthy it is.

QUALITY OF LIFE

In these pages we want to offer you tangible solutions to living a healthier life. If being one of the world's half a million centenarians is your goal, we will offer you steps to achieve it. If taking better care of yourself and living in Ultimate Health is important to you, we can offer guidelines to make that become a reality.

Together, we've collectively coached thousands of people to live their very best lives—and in the pages to follow, we want to coach you to do the same. The steps to *Ultimate Health* aren't complex. It's about developing the daily habits that work for you and your body; and keeping your mind, body, and emotional life operating at the highest level of excellence.

Your Real Age

Ultimate Health includes managing the way you age. In the pages to follow we are going to challenge you to think differently about your current age as well as provide strategies for how to improve the quality of your years. This is about more than just your chronological age. We believe there are at least three types of aging: chronological, mental, and physical. You can't stop the first one but you can take steps today to positively alter the physical and mental aging process. *Chronological*: this is your biological age. *Mental*: how young you think and feel. *Physical*: this is the level of activity you're able to participate in, your energy level, and how well your body is working.

Do you feel stressed, overloaded, sluggish, or overweight? Are you lacking sleep, hormones, or nutrients that properly fuel your brain and body and support your immune system? If you do, it's time to pay attention to the warning signs.

Research has proven that you can positively influence your current physical aging process with diet, body chemistry management, exercise, and preventive activities. You can start developing a healthier mind-set, habits, and lifestyle that will alter your mind, body, and energy.

Ultimate Health isn't just a catchy phrase a publisher made up. It's a philosophy that applies to your life. Ultimately, your health is in your hands.

But Ultimate Health is not a choice you make one day and forget about the next. It's not a diet or a decision; it's a lifestyle. Once you commit to the pursuit of Ultimate Health, you will be amazed by how much better you feel and perform. That positive reinforcement is what leads to a lifestyle that becomes second nature to maintain.

Clarity

One of the things each one of us is absolutely convinced of is the concept of holistic, preventive wellness. Holistic refers to your whole life—body, mind, and spirit. **Prevention** refers to the process of taking an active role in your health to reduce the onset of disease and ensure you live the highest quality life possible. It involves taking the necessary measures, tests, and checkups at the right time to prevent disease or diagnose it early, and to live well. The Cooper Clinic of Dallas for many years has provided world class preventive medicine evaluation with the primary goal of preventing heart disease and cancer.

If disease is diagnosed early enough, there are medical advancements necessary to fight and reverse it. Breast cancer, for instance, is a common cancer. Yet it is treatable and possible to eliminate if diagnosed in time. Similarly, heart disease, a leading killer of Americans, can be treated and even prevented, and so can other illnesses, such as diabetes.

Are you willing to change your mind-set to commit to a lifestyle of prevention? Some books are simply informational, but we hope this one can help save your life. Make the commitment today toward a lifestyle of prevention.

LIFESTYLE

Your lifestyle consists of your beliefs and priorities combined with your daily habits.

One of the reasons we wanted to write this book is to encourage you to achieve complete clarity on what kind of lifestyle you want to live. Perhaps you are reading this because there is something you want to give up, such as tobacco, alcohol, or even sugar. Or maybe you just want to lose a few pounds, slow down aging, or adopt a healthier diet. Congratulations! You are at an important crossroads in your life!

This is a book about *you*. We want to help you change bad habits, uncover good ones, and adopt a healthier lifestyle—today.

No matter what kind of life you live or what your health goals may be, research proves that exercise is one of the best ways to promote health and even slow the aging process.

Ultimate Health VIPs

1. Your lifestyle determines your longevity.
2. Exercise is medicine.
3. There are three types of aging: chronological, mental, and physical. Ultimate Health includes managing the way you age.
4. Research suggests that you can alter the effects of aging with diet, exercise, and preventive tests.
5. Making time in your busy schedule for exercise and stress relief/relaxation is paramount.

Chapter 2
Mental Management

What goes on in your mind truly impacts your health. Assess your own self-talk, your daily attitude, and your beliefs about life. Understand your outlook. Is it positive? Adopt a willingness to release grudges and forgive while focusing on the positives. Filter the input you receive from sources such as news, media, and negative people.

Ultimate Health is about achieving success in multiple areas of your life— mentally, physically, emotionally, spiritually, and even financially. Although we cover weight loss, nutrition, and food intake in the chapters ahead, living a healthy life is about more than just what you eat and absorb into your body. It is also about what you think, let go of, and refuse to believe. In this chapter we want to focus on the link between your mental outlook and your physical health. Your mind and body are intertwined, and what goes in one affects the other.

Ultimate Health for your mind includes being conscious about eliminating toxins such as unproductive thought patterns, unhealthy habits, and negative and self-limiting beliefs; and increasing positive thoughts, energy, and momentum. It encompasses being intentional about who you spend time with because the people around you greatly impact your success.

Ultimate Health is an active process of developing essential daily habits that are restorative and transformative—habits that lead to a vibrant, energetic life for decades to come.

Ultimate Health is an active process of developing essential daily habits that are restorative and transformative—habits that lead to a vibrant, energetic life for decades to come.

Have you ever known someone who attracts people, positions, things, and business opportunities to them like a magnet? Everything they touch seems to turn to gold because they are vibrant and energetic. They ooze positivity. They're inspirational and energizing. Strangers are drawn to them and their friends would do anything for them. These people emit positive energy and are so nice to be around that you want to say "yes" when they ask you to do something with them.

On the other side of the coin are the people who always seem to have a negative opinion about things. When you present a new idea, they tend to be critical or point out all the reasons why it can't be done.

They are no fun at all to be around, they miss out on opportunities, and they blame others for their failures.

Which one would you rather be around, or do business and life with? The answer is obvious, of course. People want to be around people who lift them up and encourage them to reach their goals and dreams. They inspire others to reach higher levels.

Negative people are dream killers. They give reasons why something cannot be done and often delay taking action on their own dreams as well. Their self-talk is negative and their talk to others is negative. You will often find that this negative internal self-talk builds into bitterness, anger, or self-defeating actions and beliefs. Sometimes it creates a toxic mix of feelings that lead to stress, illness, depression, or other ailments. But at other times it's more subtle. If you've ever lived with a dream-killer, you might find yourself putting your own dreams on hold just because it seems too difficult to convince them to go along with you. Are you a dream-maker, or a dream killer? Do you inspire or defeat?

What goes on in your mind impacts your health.

Think of the process of managing your mind-set the same way you think of managing your business. If you owned a company, you wouldn't leave clutter all over the front office for your clients to see. The clutter would give an appearance of disarray, distraction, and disorganization. Why, then, would you want that in your personal space? There are ways to elevate your mind-set on a daily basis to continually remind you of the positives in your life—but this takes intention.

One of the strategies Tony uses to elevate his outlook is to surround himself with positive images and affirmations. He suggests putting photographs or objects in your office or home that remind you of positive moments, achievements, and memories. Be intentional about every photograph and every space—even down to what is in each photo. Each one should keep positive thoughts flowing. Keep your environment clear of unpaid bills or other unnecessary reminders of the negative aspects of life that can clutter your mind. Leave those details for administrative days so they are not sapping your creativity, production, or focus.

Another important factor to a positive mind-set is to keep healthy people in your space. We become like those around us, so spend time with quality individuals. Vow to make every room you enter a happier space simply because you are there! Make sure you are one of those people who others feed off of to authentically improve their self-confidence, their life, and their success; doing so will also impact your own.

There are three kinds of people in this world:

Energy-givers

Energy-users

Energy-takers

Which ones do you associate with? If you hang out with energy-takers, you can bet you're being depleted more often than you're being charged up.

When you intentionally manage your mental energy and increase the positive things you think about, you inspire others to do the same.

> When you intentionally manage your mental energy and increase the positive things you think about, you inspire others to do the same.

Managing your mental health is a critical part of success. Live your life with an intentional pursuit for happiness, peace, and a positive way of thinking to reduce stress and remain balanced.

Ultimate Health VIPs

1. Mental management is a crucial aspect of Ultimate Health.
2. You are what you think! Think positive, healthy thoughts and affirmations.
3. Be intentional; surround yourself with positive people, images, places, and things to increase your mental health, outcomes, and results.
4. Continually learn and grow to develop your mind and soul. Consistently add new experiences and inspiration to your world.
5. Make every room you enter a happier place in part because you are there.

Chapter 3
Ultimate Longevity

Do you have a team of health professionals on your side?
Family doctor? Nutritionist? Dentist?
Do you have regular checkups and blood work performed?
Do your daily habits and behaviors align with real health?

You can live to be 100. That may seem like a bold statement, but it's true.

There are currently tens of thousands of people over one hundred alive on this earth. Will you be one of them?

You can live an active, healthy, and vibrant life as a centenarian or even super centenarian, depending upon how dedicated you are to achieving Ultimate Health and reversing the effects of aging.

How long do you think you will live?

Do you have a preconceived notion about your number of years on earth? When we polled people with this question, most gave a figure somewhere in the 70s. Because the average lifespan for men and women is in the mid-seventies, most people have a belief that centers around that number. But the truth is that many people live much, much longer. Others die much younger from diseases that could have been prevented and controlled.

If you take on a thoughtful and active role in your own well-being, and have regular wellness screenings, you should expect to live longer—and stronger—than the average American. The benefits are too important to ignore, because the quality of your remaining decades is largely dependent on your physical health.

> If you start now, you can create a plan for Ultimate Health that extends far beyond the normal human lifespan and increases the quality of your years above all else.

Truths About Aging

We want to shift your paradigm about what it means to grow old. Aging can be an amazing process and not a destructive one. You can literally thrive, start a new chapter in your life, and challenge yourself to new limits. You do not have to waste away in a nursing home; nor do you have to become frail in mind and body. You can age gracefully, continue to learn new things, and take on a new hobby, sport, or career, even if others around you have stopped moving, dreaming, and doing! Your life can be completely different than the average person. You can move into your next decades with vitality, and an anything-is-possible mind-set.

> You can extend your longevity by adding cardiovascular fitness, building your immune system, and acting and thinking differently.

Add Years to Your Life, and Life to Your Years

Centenarians exist in all parts of the world. At one time, some people believed it was the Mediterranean diet, rich in olive oil and red wine, that led to longevity; then, others attributed it to the high fish diet common to the Japanese. But centenarians aren't just clustered in Japan and Italy; the United States certainly has its share. In a culture of obesity, disease, and diabetes, we still have plenty of people living to the age of one hundred (and beyond!).

A supercentenarian is someone who lives beyond the age of 110 years. Imagine if you've got that much time left. What is it you'll plan to do with your life? If you remain in good health, you'll be able to travel, read, journal, listen to music, spend time with family and friends, watch movies, and learn about new things. The opportunities are endless.

The countries with the highest number of supercentenarians are believed to be the United States, United Kingdom, Japan, France, and Italy. To date, there are seven undisputed cases of people who have lived to 116 years of age or older, and the oldest verified human was Jeanne Calment, who died in 1997 at the age of 122. This is far beyond the average life span in the seventies.

There are a variety of things that contribute to preventive medicine. It is important to be aware of major family health history diseases that could compromise your future health. If you know you have a predisposition toward heart disease, for instance, you would be more inclined to watch your cholesterol, blood pressure, stop smoking, lower stress, and watch your diet.

Here are just a few ways to decrease your chances for disease and live a long and healthy life:

- Have a primary care physician and get regular checkups.
- Have interval first-class *preventive medicine* evaluations at The Cooper Clinic–Dallas or a similar reputable medical facility.
- Get your preventive blood work done at least once a year.
- Get a health team around you for all aspects of your holistic health— mind, body, and spirit.

- Follow a nutritionist's or registered dietitian's plan for eliminating the wrong foods and infusing your body and cells with nutrient-dense foods to fight aging and decrease the risk of obesity and chronic disease.
- Add stretching and balance exercises and intellectual stimulation to your anti-aging plan.

The difference between health care (preventive medicine) and sick care (going to the doctor after you feel bad) is testing, prevention, and a holistic mind-set about your health. Although most people believe they are involved in their health care, it really is *health carelessness* when you wait until you feel pain or sickness to go and try to find a solution!

Think about it. You have to maintain a high-performance vehicle to make it last longer and perform better. If you had a car you loved, you would treat it with care. You would get your oil changed properly—and at the right time—and you would make sure the transmission had the right level of fluid. You would take whatever steps necessary to protect the engine and prevent potential catastrophe. Yet many people fail to treat their bodies with equal care. They simply wait until there is pain somewhere to visit a doctor. Unfortunately, that is often too late for optimum health.

As a general rule, it is almost always easier—and less expensive—to prevent disease than it is to treat it once health is lost.

We want to show you what is possible. We want to shift your mind-set about the aging process and show you that you have more control over aging than you think. We wrote this book because we believe in health care, not "sick care." We all know and practice firsthand the concept of having a team of trained professionals that gives you insight into all areas of your life. Having a team that acts as a strong support system to help you stay ahead of the curve is a major step toward disease management.

Ultimate Health VIPs

1. You can live healthier, and longer than the average American.
2. The difference between healthcare and sick care is proactive testing, prevention, and a holistic mind-set. Be smart and proactive; work to maintain your health.
3. Look and feel ten years younger with disease prevention, screening, and developing an Ultimate Health plan with your health team.
4. Get your preventive blood work analyzed at least once a year and make adjustments where needed.

CHAPTER 4

ELIMINATING STRESS

Are you managing anxiety and making a conscious effort to eliminate stress? Is your life aligned with your values? Have you set up harmony in your home, office, and life so that things run as smoothly as possible? Is your pace of life contributing to or detracting from your overall well-being?

One of the major causes of disease, aging, and death is stress. Stress occurs when our mental, physical, or spiritual challenges exceed our ability to cope with them.

Stress kills—literally. It causes your body to secrete hormones (cortisol and adrenaline) that can have a negative impact on your health.

How Stress Destroys Lives

Your adrenal gland produces several hormones, one of which is cortisol, a stress-related hormone. A little is good, but an excess is not. If your adrenal glands secrete the hormone too much and too often, it has negative impact down the road. Examples include increased tissue inflammation, elevated blood pressure, and decreased immunity.

We do not want to teach you how to simply manage stress, but rather how to virtually eliminate it from your life. When you can reduce stress from your day, everything flows much more smoothly. Your business life, your relationships, and your physical well-being will all improve. Stress can be situational and caused by several factors, including how we plan, react, and cope with what we allow in our lives.

There will always be obstacles and issues in life that are outside your control. But those are externally driven, isolated events. Stress is what happens when pressure builds in the gap between the things we want to do and the things we are actually doing. It results from a lack of congruence between the life you want—your goals—and the life you live. For instance, if your goal is to live a debt-free life, but instead you have mountains of credit card bills rolling in, you will experience stress as a consequence. If you are constantly rushing around, always late for meetings, kids' sports activities, or church, you are creating stress during the process of getting to and from events—instead of enjoying the journey.

The best way to cure stress is to drill down to the source of the problem, and cut stress out before it even happens.

If you do a "life audit" and make a list of the top ten most stressful things that happen on a daily basis, you will begin to discover a lot of habits and processes—or lack thereof—that could be modified. By changing certain habits, you can eliminate most sources of stress in your life.

It is easy to complicate your life with so many things to be accomplished that you end up forfeiting the freedom of simplicity. We are not suggesting you become a monk, but simplifying your life will inevitably lead to a lot less stress. **Your *true* wealth is determined by the amount of things you do not**

have to worry about. Worry is a stressor.

> The best way to cure stress is to drill down to the source of the problem, and cut stress out before it even happens.

THE POWER OF MARGIN TIME

Often, the most frequent stressor in anyone's life is a lack of time. If you have ever rushed around looking for your car keys on the way to an important meeting, you know the anxiety it creates. But when you drill down to the core of the issue, you see that a *lack* of time is not actually producing the stress—it is the way you are *managing* your time. In that moment of rushing, you are stressed because you have a lack of time. But in the moments leading up to it, you had plenty.

Building margin time into your life right now—today!—is one of the fastest ways to eliminate stress. Another reason to build in margin time is to make room for life's unexpected events. When you have extra time you can accept an interruption with grace, talk to an old friend who calls at the last minute, or help someone in need. Without built-in margin time, you will feel pressed and stressed.

Other actions you can take to reduce stress in your life are:
- Eradicate disorganization
- Eliminate unnecessary commitments
- Stop procrastinating
- Let go
- Be on time
- Eliminate toxic people, places, and things
- Reduce unnecessary obligations
- Stop taking responsibility for things that are not your responsibility
- Say "no" more intentionally and strategically

Stress-related impact on your health is not always readily apparent. Sometimes it takes years or even decades before you feel the consequences of stress. The compound effect of negative influences add up each day. Ultimate

Health involves reducing stress today—for a better life tomorrow!

SELF-TALK

One of the most important concepts related to stress is to make a habit of asking yourself, "Does it really matter?" Establishing and maintaining positive self-talk that helps you diffuse stress is a good strategy for success. This practice involves body awareness as well as understanding your mind, your chemical imbalances, your hormones, and the way you live and feel. When you face a daily challenge, ask yourself if it really matters in the long term. Manage your obstacles and put things in perspective. Don't create drama or make them larger than they are. Everyone's life has challenges.

Another source of stress is incongruence. That means that something in your life isn't lining up. You think one way, but act another. Or you have a belief system about one thing, but your life represents the opposite.

When you do things that are incongruent with your core values, you will feel the serious consequences of stress. Be intentional about designing your own life, and be cautious not to overdo it in any phase of your life or to stress yourself too much mentally, emotionally, physically, or financially. Achieving congruence provides you with Ultimate Health integrity.

> Be intentional about designing your own life and be cautious not to "overdo it" in any phase of your life that stress yourself too much mentally, emotionally, physically, or financially.

COMPLETION

Completion is a significant factor when it comes to stress. When you complete projects, you feel satisfied, knowing you have accomplished something. When you have a lack of completion, you feel less peace because you're thinking about the things you need to do.

Have you ever felt stressed by a messy environment or work space? If you have projects on your desk in various stages of completion, there exists in your mental space a little part of every project still undone. You will find your mind fragmented as you think about several things you have left to do. It's important to know what your tolerance is for incompletion. If it stresses you to have things undone, make it your goal not to multitask, but to tackle one project at a time and see each one through to completion.

DOING TOO MUCH AT ONCE

Unrealistic compromise is defeating to the soul. Refuse to take on things you do not want to, things that would solely be an attempt to please other people. If you do not, you will likely find yourself stretched in too many directions. Just say no! Don't fear missed opportunities. Say no to things you're not completely sure you want to do or things that aren't going to help propel you toward your goals.

HOW DO I LIVE A LESS STRESSFUL LIFE?

Having complete clarity about what you want is the first step toward getting it. So the best way to release stress from your life is to identify stressors. Take five minutes to make a list of the things that stress you the most. Once you know what they are, you can take steps to eliminate them. To eliminate stress you must first identify the stress, its cause, and the negative habits you need to change. Make a quick hit list of the things that stress you.

Examples:
- Being late
- Over-committing
- Disorganization
- Financial actions
- Messes
- Wrong people around you
- Incomplete projects
- Saying yes to everything

Understanding the biggest stressors in your life is a great first step toward freedom away from them.

Ultimate Health VIPs

1. Your true wealth is determined by the amount of things you do not have to worry about.
2. Identify your stressors . . . then begin eliminating them!
3. Detox your life from negative people, places, and things.
4. Create systems for organization, values clarification, and completion.
5. Build margin time into your days, schedules, and calendaring.
6. When issues arise, ask yourself often, "does it really matter?" Calm down, breathe, and relax.

Chapter 5

Strengthening Your Immune System

Your immune system is a protective mechanism that detects potential harm and helps your body react. Take action to strengthen and support your immune system by eating nutritious foods that support immune health. Ask yourself if you're resting when you should, if you're washing your hands properly, protecting your body against harmful bacteria, and maintaining good hygiene.

Your body was created with an amazing immune system that fights disease and protects you in several ways. This complex network of cells, tissues, and organs works together to protect your body. Most people remain unaware of immune system dysfunction until they feel sick or get blood test results that show some abnormality.

The immune system includes visible barriers like the skin, eyes, nose, and mouth, as well as invisible barriers that fight infection. The lymph system detects bacteria and waste. The lymph nodes can become swollen if an infection exists in the body. They contain lymphocytes that trap germs and destroy them.

Your immune system has the incredible ability to:

- Detect bacteria and viruses that manage to get into the body—before they have a chance to reproduce.
- Eliminate viruses or bacteria that have already reproduced.
- Create a barrier that prevents bacteria and viruses from entering your body.
- Fight against the development of cancerous cells.

The Science of Life

Vaccines against microorganisms that cause diseases can prepare the body's immune system and help fight or prevent an infection. Even though the immune system is an invisible internal bodily system, how well it functions determines your aging, health, and activity. Most people are unaware that there are active steps that can be taken in order to improve the overall health of the immune system.

The most important elements of the immune system that are improved by immunization are T cells and B cells (along with the antibodies they produce). Memory B cells and memory T cells attack foreign molecules that the body has previously encountered.

Minimize Stress to Increase Immunity

In the previous chapter we discussed stress and the harmful effect it has on overall health and longevity, and this bears repeating: stress kills. Eliminating the stressful people, places, and things in your daily life will work wonders for your overall wellness and for your physical, emotional, and intellectual health. Make a habit of minimizing stressful emotions.

Some of the most effective immune-boosting activities are:

- Exercise daily.
- Meditate, pray, and detox your life.
- Reduce fat and sugar consumption.
- Maintain a diet rich in antioxidants.
- Wash your hands often and keep your environment clean.

Exercise Daily

Getting active with regular, daily exercise is one of the best ways to boost your immune system. Cardiovascular exercise increases cells that fight infection; so even a brisk walk or jog is beneficial. When you increase your heart rate you get an infusion of endorphins to fight stress and, along with them, a flood of mood-enhancing chemicals.

> Getting active with regular, daily exercise is one of the best ways to boost your immune system.

Reduce Fat and Sugar Consumption

Fats and sugars create stress on the immune system, while nutritious foods rich in antioxidants, vitamins, and nutrients can boost immunity and help fight infection.

Vitamins B, C, D, E, and zinc all provide an immune boost. The best ways to get them are through foods rich in antioxidants such as berries, kiwi, apples, kale, onions, spinach, sweet potatoes, garlic, carrots, peppers, and other brightly colored fruits and vegetables. Your body produces free radicals, which are molecules that can damage cells. Antioxidants help neutralize free radicals to prevent them from doing damage, and researchers believe that when the balance between free radicals and antioxidants is upset, it can contribute to developing cancer, heart disease, and other age-related diseases.

Take the steps necessary to boost your immune system. Be aware of this vital system within your body as you age, and work to develop and strengthen it.

ULTIMATE HEALTH VIPS

1. Reduce stress to strengthen your immune system.
2. Research, become aware of, and choose immune system-boosting foods!
3. Vaccines against microorganisms that cause diseases may prepare the body's immune system and help fight—or prevent—an infection.
4. Utilize meditation, music, prayer, and anything else that positively contributes to your spiritual and emotional well-being in order to help boost your body's natural immune system (including proper rest).
5. Wash your hands often and keep your environment as clean as possible.
6. Maintaining cardiovascular fitness through regular exercise has been shown to be a significant immune booster.

Exercise: Write down 3 things you will commit to that will strengthen your health.

1.

2.

3.

Chapter 6
Preventive Testing

Early detection of an illness can save your life. Stay current on screenings, blood work reviews, EKGs, MRIs, hormone testing, urinalysis, mammograms, and any other pertinent preventive tests. Knowledge is power!

Each year medical organizations, hospitals, and physician groups promote the importance of annual testing such as mammograms, skin cancer detection, dental visits, blood work exams, and physicals. But the question is: are you *living* it? In this chapter we want to explore common routine testing vital to managing your health.

The Basic Physical

In your annual checkup, your physical will evaluate things like reflexes, blood pressure, your heart sounds, and basic blood tests that check your cholesterol levels.

Other tests include:

- EKG
- Treadmill stress test
- CT scan
- Blood tests - Thyroid, Vitamin D, Omega 3
- Colonoscopy
- Gynecological exam
- Prostate testing
- Hormone levels
- Dental checkup
- Full body skin cancer screening

CIMT - A New Weapon Against America's Most Notorious Killer

Mickie Sallmander, MS, certified vascular sonographer, points out that heart disease claims one American life every 37 seconds, over twice the rate of all cancers combined. Still, it remains a highly preventable disease. The CIMT test can detect early signs of atherosclerosis, the underlying cause of heart attack and stroke, before any symptoms appear.

In this age of health awareness and medical testing it seems unfathomable that heart disease can afflict so many and strike with such stealth. Yet two-thirds of women and half of all men who die from heart attack show no prior symptoms. This may be because tests like Angiograms and EKGs detect a problem only after significant arterial blockage has occurred.

The 15 minute CIMT test uses FDA approved software and holds an advantage over more expensive and intrusive procedures because it can assess heart risk before plaque accumulates in the arteries, and does not require undressing, exercising or drawing blood.

CIMT stands for Carotid Intima-Media Thickness and measures the first two layers of the carotid artery. The thicker the arterial wall, the greater the risk for heart attack or stroke.

While the CIMT itself has been used in clinical studies for over 18 years, the CIMT test can now calculate a "vascular age" in comparison to one's chronological age based on the thickness of the carotid artery. By this measure a 46 year old with a vascular age twenty years above her chronological age shares the same risk for heart attack or stroke as a 66 year old.

Results from the CIMT test has been published in JAMA, NEJM, Lancet, Circulation and Stroke, with articles citing results from large clinical trials where thousands of people were tested. The American Heart Association recommends CIMT as a safe, inexpensive and accurate predictor of future cardiovascular events.

The test can be performed in an office environment and analyzes the findings to create a user-friendly risk report so patients can understand the results along with their doctors. Steps can then be taken to halt or even reverse the damage.

However, many potential CIMT test candidates—people age 40 and above without any symptoms—fail to receive the message before it's too late. Preventative tests like the CIMT test are doubly important for individuals with traditional red flags such as family history of heart disease, weight problems, high cholesterol or high blood pressure, and diabetes.

The CIMT test is less time consuming than giving blood and feels the same as having a sonogram. "I lost my brother to heart disease," says Paul, 51, a CIMT test patient. "He was only 42. So for me, taking 15 minutes on a lunch break to potentially add 20 years to my life seems like time well spent."

Family History—and Why It Matters

You have likely heard about the importance of DNA as it relates to preventive medicine and the quest for Ultimate Health. But it can be difficult to wade through what is really important. Should DNA testing be a part of your health management plan? Or should you forego it altogether?

In some families, there are generations of specific types of cancer incidence; so specific testing to determine if you're at risk may help with prevention and understanding risk factors and treatments. DNA is important, but how critical is it to understand risk factors and family history? Before we answer that question, let's take a look at what DNA really is.

DNA is the blueprint of biological life. It is not only responsible for transferring hereditary information from generation to generation, it is also relevant for today's inherent workings in the body. DNA controls the production of proteins and determines the structure of a cell. It is the foundation of your body.

Since DNA duplicates itself at cell division, the genetic information gets passed down from one generation to another. Doctors and scientists have studied the value of this information for years. Genetic testing that identifies changes in chromosomes, genes, or proteins can uncover an inherited disorder or an individual at high risk for certain cancers and diseases.

Understanding your genetic profile can arm you with information you need to maximize your health potential. If, for instance, you knew your family history contained a predisposition for cardiovascular disease, you would be inclined to develop a regimen focused on reducing risk. You would eat fewer fatty foods; you would exercise more and in a manner that strengthened your heart, and you would get a CIMT test.

The results of your genetic testing may help to:
• Diagnose a disease
• Find gene changes responsible for an already diagnosed disease
• Assess how severe a disease might be
• Guide selection of medicines and other treatments
• Find gene changes that increase the risk of developing a disease
• Find gene changes that could be passed on to children

Every human is genetically unique—even identical twins. In addition, our genes determine our body's response to the foods we eat, the physical activity we take part in, the way we manage stress, and many other factors.

Scientists have studied the importance of understanding the interaction between our genes and our lifestyle choices—such as exercise, foods, medicine, and nutrition—and how, for Ultimate Health, we can modify and work with what we have been given. *You cannot change your genes, but you can maximize your health and wellness through more positive and customized lifestyle choices.* Do you need genetic testing? We believe that is your own personal choice. You need awareness of the diseases that run in your family, and then consider testing yourself if colon or breast cancer or other diseases run in your family.

Ultimately, you must understand your own body, develop a passion for knowledge, and maintain health patterns and fitness levels. Work with your physician to determine what you are most at risk for and what kinds of tests are best for you. Live each day in wellness to reduce the probability of disease.

Ultimate Health VIPs

1. Preventive testing saves—and extends—lives.
2. You can live as though you were physically many years younger simply through early detection, planning, and troubleshooting in order to prevent disease.
3. Know your numbers! Get your cholesterol, hormones, and blood tested annually and as often as optimal for Ultimate Health maintenance.
4. Sharing your family history with your health team can help to assess risk factors and formulate a proactive plan.

CHAPTER 7

EXERCISE, MOVEMENT, AND LONGEVITY

Physical exercise matters and it should be regular, frequent, and ongoing. Strength resistance, cardiovascular exercise (aerobics), balance, and stretching all promote a better-operating body.

An exercise fitness study of 13,000 men and women from the world-renowned Cooper Clinic in Dallas was published in 1989, in *The Journal of the American Medical Association* (JAMA) showing that individuals with the lowest levels of fitness suffered more than twice the death rate of those with just a moderate level of fitness. It validated the truth that the risk for all causes of mortality and serious disease, including heart disease, cancer, and diabetes, is lowered by being physically fit.

Daily exercise can turn back the hands of time. Just thirty minutes of sustained activity, most days of the week can literally change or even save your life! That's a remarkable thought, but it's true. If you can add thirty minutes of movement to your day, you will transform your health. It's the healthy habits you create that matter. Habits add up in a compound effect to give us the individual outcome we create. Undeniably, decades of research shows that exercise, eating healthy, and maintaining proper weight are the three most important habits you can adopt to enhance longevity.

Studies have proven that a lack of cardiovascular fitness through regular exercise is linked with high blood pressure, obesity, diabetes, heart disease, and strokes, in addition to increased stress, cancer, and other disease states that shorten life. The science is there. Exercise heals.

> The risk for most causes of death and serious disease—including heart disease, cancer, and diabetes—is lowered by being physically fit.

The unexercised body begins to fall apart after a certain age, slowly declining at around 30 or so. Scientific studies clearly demonstrate that if you do not exercise you could face:
- steady loss of bone mass
- gradual loss of protective muscle mass
- decline in aerobic capacity (endurance)
- lower energy levels
- impaired physical functioning
- weakened immune function
- loss of mental functioning

The good news is that much of your aging is within your control. If you add exercise to your daily regimen, you'll become stronger and healthier.

The goal, as Drs. Ken and Tyler Cooper state in their book, *Start Strong, Finish Strong*, is to "square off the curve" of life by enjoying your greatest possible levels of strength, stamina, and mental acumen right up to your final breath. The first step toward doing this is to eliminate the self-limiting beliefs you may have concerning fitness. In this chapter, we hope to create awareness of the myths about fitness that may have affected your beliefs about how you live your life. Chances are that you have believed one or more of the myths below, even though absolutely none of them are correct.

Myth #1: I do not need to exercise. I just need vitamins and a healthy body weight to be fit.

Myth #2: Exercise requires a gym membership and takes too much time.

Myth #3: Exercise-based fitness provides no protection against the ravages of aging. It's all about heredity.

In his work at the Cooper Clinic, Dr. Wilson has witnessed firsthand the positive lifestyle benefits that exercise and fitness combined with caloric restriction bring to his patients. When patients decided to increase their daily movement and activity, it positively impacted their work life, mental state, and personal relationships.

How much exercise does it take to reach just the minimal level of fitness? The answer: very little. If you already walk a lot during your day, jog or run! Refuse to place limits on what you can achieve. We have seen 80-year-old women run full marathons and elderly men at the gym lifting more weight than teenagers. Begin slowly and heed the advice of your physician. Even the completely sedentary person can start at an easy 20-25 minutes per mile pace for two miles, five times a week, and dramatically increase longevity and vigor.

Get started today. There is simply no reason for you to not get out there and jog, run, walk, or bike—as long as your physician says it is okay. Though this is not a weight loss book, it's still worth pointing out that exercise is the fastest way to shed extra pounds. One of the catalysts for this book was the transformation Tony had when he started eliminating sugar and other unhealthy foods, monitoring calories, and focusing on a fitness regimen. He had never really been an exercise freak or fitness guru, but each time he met with a successful client through the years to coach them on excellence in their business life, he could see how their physical fitness, (or lack of it) was negatively impacting them. If you're unhealthy, your personal and business life suffers because you're not as strong mentally or physically to multitask and operate with excellence. Nutrition, oxygen, circulation, balance, and fitness are all contributors to being as sharp as you can be. When Tony decided to research and gain knowledge to understand all he could, his own life changed.

"It's amazing now when people don't recognize me, because in my old photos, I looked so much heavier. I was never overweight, but today people tell me I look ten years younger, and I certainly feel it," Tony says. "I began educating myself on hormones, metabolism issues, and exercise, and I started seeing the huge impact it had on vitality, aging well, and Ultimate Health. All that research led me to partner with the other authors of this book, and it also revealed some powerful truths:

- Exercise can lower your blood pressure
- Exercise can lower your risk of heart disease
- Exercise can improve your mental and emotional health
- Exercise is 'nature's best tranquilizer' for stress reduction
- Exercise can improve your sex life
- Exercise can extend the life of those with adult-onset diabetes
- Weight-bearing exercise will counteract bone loss that occurs with aging and sedentary lifestyles
- Exercise improves your balance and decreases your risk of injuries from falls
- Exercise (even just walking) can improve your immunity
- Exercise can lower your risk of getting cancer.

Effects of Fitness on Aging

With a regular fitness program, you can hold the effects of aging at bay. Age-related decline will be slower in those who stay fit versus those who neglect their bodies. Today, Tony's focus on fitness has trickled down to his employees. One has lost more than thirty pounds! Now it's not uncommon to see them walking during the day, exercising between meetings, or having actual meetings during a workout session. It's incredibly rewarding to witness a culture getting healthier.

> With a regular fitness program, you can reduce effects of aging. Age-related decline will be slower in those who stay fit versus those who neglect their bodies.

Your Heart Health

Your aerobic fitness and cardiovascular conditioning has been proven by medical researchers to play a major role in both QOL (quality of life) and POL (prolongation of life).

Regular moderate exercise conditions our bodies in ways that help reduce and control the risk for obesity, insulin resistance (diabetes), heart disease, hypertension, cancer, and stress-related illnesses.

Drs. Kenneth and Tyler Cooper strategically employ the following Keys to Preventive Health Excellence at The Cooper Clinic:

- *Evaluation* of health status through superior history and physical, targeted blood work, treadmill stress testing, rapid CT scanning, colonoscopy, skin cancer screening, and individualized additional organ testing as indicated
- *Education* on preventive health tactics for exercise, nutrition, stress reduction, and skin cancer prevention
- *Motivation* by in-depth discussion with individual specialists in key areas of concern
- *Implementation for effectiveness* as discussed with your physician in a thorough one-on-one debriefing
- *Program reevaluation and maintenance* at selected intervals

The primary goals of this approach are two-fold: first, **prevent** heart disease and cancer if possible; and if not, **diagnose** heart disease and cancer early enough to stop them.

Essential Preventive Health Strategies

Prevention can save your life.

The American Institute for Cancer Research reports that you and I can help **prevent one-third of cancers** by lifestyle changes such as limiting alcohol, controlling weight, and exercising regularly. In fact, if you can limit alcohol altogether, do. You could lower your risk for cancers of the GI tract and breast cancer in women.

According to the American Cancer Society, nine of the top ten cancer killers are related to obesity. Other key factors relating to cancer are:

• Obesity – Smoking – Inactivity – Alcohol – Vitamin D deficiency

In the case of the most common cancer, skin cancer, excessive unprotected sun exposure plays the key role. One person dies every hour from melanoma. It's a deadly skin cancer, so sun protection is one of the key habits to prevention.

The primary habits you can adopt in your own life to slow the effects of aging are:

• Stop smoking
• Correct/prevent obesity
• Eliminate inactivity
• Get your blood levels tested
• Control stress
• Increase sun protection to reduce damage

Cardiovascular fitness is an excellent preventive health strategy.

Hard proof exists in recently published peer-reviewed medical literature that cardiorespiratory fitness (CRF) is a trustworthy predictor of both longevity and quality of life (QOL). These respected studies span three decades of life. Here are a few facts:

• Your level of CRF, as measured by treadmill stress testing, is a proven predictor of death risk, longevity, and QOL in the near, intermediate, and long term. Low CRF is routinely associated with high death rates at earlier ages, not merely from sedentary lifestyle but also due to accompanying risk factors such as obesity, diabetes, and hypertension.

- Medicare-aged individuals who maintain CRF have been recently shown to experience 30 percent lower health expenditures!

Do You Need to Start Exercising?

How fast a person walks is a good predictor of longevity. If you can walk 3.5 mph for one mile, you have a high probability of longer life, commonly well beyond 80 years of age.

A cardiovascular risk factor study, involving a quarter-million 55-to-80-year-olds, looked at the presence of risk factors and occurrence of death, heart attacks, and strokes.

Risk factors for CVD (cardiovascular disease) include: diabetes, smoking, and a blood pressure of > 120/80 and cholesterol >180. Men with two or more risk factors were six times more likely to die than those with no risk factors, and women were three times more likely to die.

You do not have to run or even walk to achieve and maintain CRF. Elliptical biking, water aerobics, and swimming are excellent substitutes.

The takeaway? Get moving, and enjoy a life of Ultimate Health.

The President's Council on Physical Fitness and Sports reports that 74 percent of American women and 66 percent of men fail to meet even the 30-minute guideline for fitness. But those people have a choice . . . and so do you.

Choose health and even though it might be inconvenient or stretch you beyond your comfort zone choose to move! Find a sport or fitness routine you are interested in and just do it! Just *thirty minutes* of movement most days of the week will lengthen your life.

Ultimate Health VIPs

1. Many overlook the fact that all four types of exercise should be in most people's routine: resistance, cardio, stretching, and balance.

2. Effective exercise is one of the single most important things you can do for your body.

3. When you engage in physical activity such as running, biking, yoga, or weight training, you increase your heart rate and can really super-turbo-charge your metabolism!

4. High-intensity interval training (like running short sprints) also boosts metabolism and requires minimal time commitment.

5. Resistance training activates muscles all over your body and increases your average daily metabolic rate. Yet another reason to pump iron!

CHAPTER 8

Oral Health

Are you brushing and flossing enough?

Going for regular checkups? Dental and oral hygiene are important factors in staying healthy.

In recent years, emerging research has shed a harsh light on the dangerous link between gum disease and heart health. Studies have revealed that a shocking *84 percent* of patients with coronary artery disease (CAD) also have periodontal disease and that this same condition significantly raises your risk of hypertension, heart attack, and severe coronary lesions.

Evidence also suggests that oral infections are capable of raising notorious inflammatory markers like C-reactive protein (CRP) and fibrinogen, both of which are major red flags for heart disease and atherosclerosis.

Meanwhile, other studies show that *half* of all patients with chronic periodontitis also have *Streptococcus mutans*—the very same bacteria found in their dental plaque—lining the walls of their arteries, too. Additionally, periodontal disease also appears to be connected to high total cholesterol and triglyceride levels, along with reduced levels of health-boosting HDL (or "good") cholesterol.

The way we maintain our teeth, gums, and mouth is more important than most people realize. Brushing our teeth every day is something we do mostly on autopilot, but there is so much more that needs to occur in order to have ultimate oral health.

Your mouth is teeming with bacteria—most of which are harmless. Normally, the body's natural defenses, along with good oral care such as daily brushing and flossing, can keep these bacteria under control. Harmful bacteria, however, can sometimes grow out of control and cause oral infections such as tooth decay and gum disease. Additionally, dental procedures, medications, or treatments that reduce saliva flow disrupt the normal balance of bacteria in your mouth, or breach the mouth's normal protective barriers, and may make it easier for bacteria to enter your bloodstream.

> Oral health can significantly impact your overall health.

Your oral health may contribute to various diseases and conditions, including:

Endocarditis. Gum disease and dental procedures that cut your gums may allow bacteria to enter your bloodstream. If you have a weak immune system or a damaged heart valve, this can cause infection in other parts of the body such as an infection of the inner lining of the heart (endocarditis).

Cardiovascular disease. Some research suggests that heart disease, clogged arteries, and stroke may be linked to oral bacteria, possibly due to chronic inflammation from periodontitis, a severe form of gum disease.

Pregnancy and childbirth. Gum disease has been linked to premature birth and low birth weight.

Diabetes. Diabetes reduces the body's resistance to infection, putting the gums at risk. Additionally, people who have inadequate blood sugar control may develop more frequent and severe infections of the gums and the bone that hold teeth in place—and may lose more teeth than do people who have good blood sugar control.

Osteoporosis. Osteoporosis, which causes bones to become weak and brittle, may be associated with periodontal bone loss and tooth loss.

- Worldwide, 60–90 percent of schoolchildren and nearly 100 percent of adults have dental cavities.
- Dental cavities can be prevented by maintaining a constant, low level of fluoride in the oral cavity.
- Severe periodontal (gum) disease, which may result in tooth loss, is found in 15–20 percent of middle-aged (35-44 years) adults.
- Globally, about 30 percent of people aged 65–74 have no natural teeth.
- Oral disease in children and adults is higher among poor and disadvantaged population groups.
- Risk factors for oral diseases include an unhealthy diet, tobacco use, harmful alcohol use, poor oral hygiene, and social determinants.

How Can I Protect My Oral Health?

To protect your oral health, resolve to practice good oral hygiene every day.
- Brush your teeth at least twice a day
- Replace your toothbrush every three to four months
- Floss daily
- Eat a healthy diet and limit between-meal snacks, especially if they're sugary
- Schedule regular dental checkups

Watch for signs and symptoms of oral disease and contact your dentist as soon as a problem arises. Remember, taking care of your oral health is an investment in your overall health.

Ultimate Health VIPs

1. Oral health can significantly impact your overall health.
2. Emerging research has shed a harsh light on the dangerous link between gum disease and heart health.
3. To protect your oral health, resolve to practice good oral hygiene every day.
4. Watch for signs and symptoms of oral disease and contact your dentist as soon as a problem arises.
5. Get regular cleanings and annual checkups.

Chapter 9
Vision Care

Most people aren't aware of how important nutrition is to eye health. Are you eating to support your eyes? The same vitamins and nutrient-rich foods that contribute to healthy skin and organs also promote eye health.

Protect your eyes from harsh sunlight and eat the foods that will help prevent cataracts later in life. Get regular eye exams. Ask yourself: do you wear eye protection when you mow or work around the house? All these factors add up to promoting ultimate eye care.

Of the five senses (sight, hearing, smell, taste, and touch), most people would place vision near the top of the senses they'd never want to lose. Yet so many people take their vision for granted. Protecting the eyes involves the same process you go through to live and maintain Ultimate Health in every other area. Positive, healthy food choices, preventive checkups, and maintenance are key.

Anything good for heart, skin, and blood vessel health is also good for your eyes!

> ### Anything good for heart, skin, and blood vessel health is also good for your eyes!

NUTRITION AND EYE HEALTH

Research shows the benefits of eating nine to ten servings of fresh (vine-ripened, uncooked) fruits and vegetables daily. While this is true for health in general, dietary discipline also contributes significantly to eye health—specifically to prevention of cataracts and macular degeneration.

Dr. Wilson's brother, ophthalmologist Gary W. Wilson, questioned 30,000 prospective Lasik surgery patients over a decade about their daily consumption of fresh fruits and vegetables. Ninety percent admitted consuming from zero to less than four servings of fresh fruits and vegetables per day. Only one in 500 responded that nine to ten servings per day were routine. While that might sound like a lot of servings, increasing your intake of organic, colorful, healthy fruits and vegetables will increase your overall health.

VITAMIN SUPPLEMENTS AND EYE HEALTH

Many believe a multivitamin takes care of their needs. However, Dr. Wilson points out that the typical multivitamin only contains up to 30 supplemental elements while the whole-food fruits and vegetables in a product like Juice Plus contain 10,000 phytonutrients, according to nutrition research. The Academy of Nutrition and Dietetics reports that foods with vitamins E, C, and A promote good eye health. It is not just about carrots.

The antioxidants in fresh fruits and vegetables cancel out the free radicals that damage our various body tissues as a result of routine daily metabolism, sun exposure, poor dietary habits, and environmental exposures. Like other parts of the body, the cornea and retina of the eye are protected by this optimal nutrition approach.

> The antioxidants in fresh fruits and vegetables cancel out the free radicals that damage our various body tissues as a result of routine daily metabolism, sun exposure, poor dietary habits, and environmental exposures.

EXERCISE AND EYE HEALTH

We all know exercise has been shown to promote brain health, function, and renewal. Since the eye (retina and optic nerve) is part of the brain, this exercise benefit has been found to extend to ocular tissues as well. Exercise for your heart health, *and* for your eyes!

INTERVAL EYE EXAMS

Eye exams should be performed on a regular basis. It is important for a child to have an exam prior to starting kindergarten. Various forms of impaired vision commonly contribute to poor classroom performance and lead to a compounding of educational problems for children when undetected. Examples include childhood glaucoma, strabismus, and astigmatism, among others.

CONTROL YOUR WEIGHT

Obesity leads to diabetes and hypertension, both of which destroy eyes, hearts, kidneys, and the brain (strokes). If you have diabetes or high blood pressure, work to control your blood sugar levels and blood pressure. Poorly controlled blood pressure can cause eye strokes and contribute to macular degeneration with eventual blindness. This is due to the effects on the key retinal vessels serving the optic nerve region at the back of the eye. *The com-*

bination of high blood pressure and poorly controlled diabetes is extremely damaging to the eye and will usually result in rapid onset of irreparable blindness. It also wreaks havoc on the kidneys, leading to the need for dialysis or kidney transplantation.

> The combination of high blood pressure and poorly controlled diabetes is extremely damaging to the eye and will usually result in rapid onset of irreparable blindness.

WEAR EYE PROTECTION

Ophthalmologists commonly see patients with fragments of steel, rock debris, whole nails, and other foreign bodies ricocheted into the eyeball with catastrophic results. Mowing the lawn or edging without protective eyewear is commonly done with tragic results as debris is kicked up into the eye at speeds of up to 200 mph. Similarly, firing rifles or shotguns may occasionally lead to blowback of damaging debris into the eye.

Other potential dangers include:

Hazardous chemicals. Handle alkali, acids, and drain-opening chemicals with eyewear. Splash-back of these chemicals will instantly and seriously damage the cornea, with serious and often permanent damage.

Blows to the eye. Fist fights, martial arts, tennis, racquetball, handball, or any concussive blow directly on the eyeball creates a shockwave effect that essentially pulverizes the retina with resultant blindness. Be cautious when opening bottles with contents under pressure! The cork on a champagne bottle seems harmless but could inflict real damage on the eye.

Contacts. Avoid ever putting contact lenses in your mouth and then putting them in your eyes. This is also true of touching infected skin (fever blisters, staph infection, etc.) and then touching the eye. Bacterial or viral transfer to the eye happens casually but sometimes leads to a tragic eye infection. Never continue wearing contacts if you think you may have pinkeye or other infection as the infectious agent may be inoculated into the cornea with serious consequences. Avoid wearing extended-wear contacts if possible, as this may lead to deficient oxygenation of the cornea, which is damaging and may predispose contact-wearers to infections they would not otherwise normally experience.

Maintaining your eye health is just as important as preventing illness or issues in other organs. One of the most important things you can do to maintain strong eye health is to eat a lot of greens and colorful vegetables that provide nutrients and vitamins to your cells.

Ultimate Health VIPs

1. Anything good for heart, skin, and blood vessel health is also good for your eyes.
2. Like other parts of the body, the cornea and retina of the eye are protected by the antioxidants in fresh fruits and vegetables; eat plenty!
3. Exercise has been shown to promote brain health, function, and renewal. Since the eye is part of the brain, this exercise benefit has been found to extend to ocular tissues as well.
4. Eye exams should be performed on an annual basis.
5. Be safe and protect your eyes with sunglasses and protection gear when working or being around dangerous activities.

CHAPTER 10

TOXIN ELIMINATION

Toxic chemicals can seep into your body through your skin, food, or the air you breathe. Toxins are potentially hazardous substances that can place an extra toll on your body and cause your liver and kidneys to work overtime as they filter fluids. (And let's not forget emotional toxins as well.) Are you protecting yourself?

What goes in affects what comes out, and what goes in also determines how well you can perform. Are you fueling your body properly with healthy, unprocessed, nutritious foods? Are you consciously avoiding the chemicals that exist in cleaning supplies, pesticides on foods, the lawn, dry cleaning, and other toxic substances?

Watching what you eat is about more than just obesity. It is also about making sure the quality of what you ingest is clean and pure. Many manufactured foods are highly processed with chemicals, and even many fruits and vegetables are treated with pesticides and harmful substances that affect the liver and other organs. Do your best to live in Ultimate Health by eliminating toxins and opting for organic foods whenever possible.

ALL FOODS ARE NOT CREATED EQUAL

The Environmental Working Group annual report listed the fruits and vegetables that ranked highest in pesticide residue. The list is called the dirty dozen for a reason. In 2012, the list included apples, celery, sweet bell peppers, peaches, strawberries, imported nectarines, grapes, spinach, lettuce, cucumbers, domestic blueberries, and potatoes. This list is an eye-opener because it illustrates how the foods we believe to be healthy may be contaminated with toxic chemicals.

So what is the solution? Buy organic. Another list exists, called the clean 15, which outlines the safest fruits and vegetables. This refers to the foods least likely to have pesticide residue. The 2012 list included onions, sweet corn, pineapples, avocado, cabbage, sweet peas, asparagus, mangoes, eggplant, kiwi, domestic cantaloupe, sweet potatoes, grapefruit, watermelon, and mushrooms.

> Do your best to live in Ultimate Health by eliminating toxins and opting for organic foods, surrounding yourself with great people, and maintaining clean environments.

ALLERGY TOXINS

Have you ever noticed a feeling of bloating, cramping, or even sudden diarrhea within a couple hours of eating? You could be one of a growing number of individuals who are suffering from sensitivities to certain common foods in their diets. Traditional medicine has focused for a long time on the 2 percent of adults and 5 percent of children in the United States who suffer from severe food allergies that cause a rash or throat swelling, but the extent of sensitivity to certain foods is becoming more and more recognized.

From 1997 to 2007, the prevalence of reported food allergy increased 18 percent among children. Food allergy reactions include the well-known fatal or near-fatal anaphylactic reaction to peanuts, tree nuts, shellfish, and occasionally milk as well as adverse reactions to toxins released from food (bacterial food poisoning).

Classic allergies to food can result in an acute onset of symptoms following ingestion of the triggering food allergen, as well as in chronic disorders such as atopic dermatitis. Reactions to these foods by an allergic person occur within minutes and can range from a tingling sensation around the lips, to hives, to even death, depending on the severity of the reaction. Foods that are most commonly implicated in triggering these allergic reactions are eggs, milk, peanuts, shellfish, tree nuts, wheat, and GMO corn. Awareness and education regarding the seriousness of food allergies is increasing, and recent studies are beginning to focus on the subtype of adverse food reactions called food sensitivity.

Food sensitivities are more common than food allergies and frequently go undiagnosed. Food sensitivities cause more of a delayed reaction after ingesting the offending food (hours to several days later). The most common offenders are gluten (wheat protein), dairy products, and nightshades (tomatoes, potatoes, eggplant, and peppers). Food sensitivity involves a different immune pathway and results in a more chronic and systemic inflammatory response. If left untreated, this can lead to end-organ damage, autoimmune disease, gastrointestinal cancer, pancreatic enzyme deficiency, and/or behavioral issues. Food sensitivities are more difficult to detect because the symptoms can be delayed and can be confused by other foods or substances that have been ingested. The most common symptoms of food sensitivity include: gas, bloating, indigestion, headaches, migraines, fatigue, lethargy, mood swings, depression, restlessness, and joint pain. Know your body, and understand what kind of foods fuel it the best.

This chapter is about eliminating toxins from your environment. Most people think of chemicals, such as cleaning supplies, pesticides on the lawn or around the home, and chemicals on foods as the biggest culprits, but emotional toxins can be just as damaging.

It is a simple saying that what goes into your body (and your mind for that matter) determines the quality of what comes out, in terms of how well you think, feel, and achieve. It's important to fuel your body well and to pay attention to what you are allowing yourself to eat, think, hear, and see. Chemical toxins exist in the food we eat, the grass we walk on, and the air we breathe. Yet the toxins we are exposed to extend beyond just the physical and chemical. Toxins can also include any negative or harmful event, thought, emotion, substance, or habit that has the potential to affect your performance or life. Emotional toxins are negative messages that stress your mind and body. Today we are all bombarded by negative messages we can't control, unless we literally turn off the technology.

The average child witnesses murders, violence, and sex each week on television. The average adult gets hundreds of solicitations, messages, emails, visual images, and advertisements sent to their minds, inboxes, and lives each week.

What you see, read, listen to, and think about each day can affect the way you perform. Working to eliminate distractions at work, for instance, helps you focus better. When you eliminate things that negatively impact your life, relationships, and business, you will find that you have much more margin time, creativity, and personal success. Identify and eliminate unproductive events, activities, and habits from your schedule.

Ultimate Health VIPs

1. Remember: chemical toxins exist in the food we eat, the grass we walk on, and the air we breathe.
2. Toxins can also include any negative or harmful event, thought, emotion, substance, or habit that has the potential to affect your performance or life.
3. Do your best to live in Ultimate Health by eliminating toxins and opting for organic foods, surrounding yourself with great people, and maintaining clean environments.
4. Do a personal audit of your life. Are there people, places, and things that need to be let go of?

Exercise: Make a list of 3 unhealthy habits, thoughts, or relationships in your life. Is it time to let go?

1.

2.

3.

Chapter 11
Hormones

A hormone is a chemical released by a cell or a gland in one part of your body that sends out messages that affect cells in other parts of your body. In essence, it's a chemical messenger that transports a signal from one cell to another. Have you tested your hormonal status (estrogen, testosterone, thyroid, DHEA, etc.)? Are you supplementing where you should?

Your body is a magnificent, complex machine. In each decade, changes occur that affect the way you live and perform. Most people do not realize that their own body is a chemical manufacturing plant. Your body makes hormones, endorphins, and other amazing chemicals that affect the balance of your mood, health, and happiness.

Here are the most common myths people believe about hormones:

Myth #1: Men don't need estrogen and women don't need testosterone.

Myth #2: Exercise and nutrition have no effect on our hormones.

Myth #3: My primary care physicians have adequate knowledge about hormones and healthy aging.

In this chapter, we want to touch on the role hormones play in your life and identify their critical functions.

Thyroid, estrogen, testosterone, and other hormones bathe the cells in our body tissues. Our endocrine (hormone) system regulates all essential functions of our bodies. It begins a decline in function at between 25 and 30 years of age. Hormones play a marvelous, intimate role in youthfulness and function. Previously, age-related decreases (endocrine decline) of various hormone levels were accepted as normal, but today there are a lot of different options to replace or stabilize hormone levels.

MISCONCEPTIONS

It is a common misconception that certain hormones are only relevant to one sex or the other. Estrogen, progesterone, and testosterone play a key function in all humans—male or female. If your hormones are out of balance, it can wreak havoc.

Testosterone is a prime example of a hormone that is commonly mistaken to be "for *men* only." But were you aware that it has significant impact as a *brain* hormone? After the age of 40, many of us start feeling the effects of aging. Symptoms of low T may include extra belly fat, mental fog, loss of muscle tone, extreme afternoon fatigue around 3-4 PM, and sleepless nights. More often than not, it is simply a function of keeping hormones in check; many of these "old age" feelings will disappear once testosterone levels are returned to normal.

Many people fail to understand the role hormones play in their physiology, but hormonal fluctuations are a big part of who we are. Estrogen and progesterone are common examples of hormones that are mistaken to be "for *women* only." Males produce progesterone in order to create testosterone and for their adrenal glands to make cortisone. Progesterone promotes normal sleep patterns, facilitates thyroid hormone function, and helps use fat for energy. Surprisingly, when low testosterone occurs, relative estrogen levels increase. Men begin to experience erectile dysfunction, the loss of muscle mass, and increased fatty tissue in the chest.

As men are dealing with Low T, women suffer from estrogen dominance. Depression, panic attacks, low self-esteem, headaches, vaginal infection, and arthritis are all common symptoms. Women in their forties are unfortunately sometimes labeled "unstable" when they have high levels of estrogen—or normal levels accompanied by low progesterone.

> Many people fail to understand the role hormones play in their physiology, but hormonal fluctuations are a big part of who we are.

Thyroid hormone is most easily related to both sexes and regulates metabolic energy. If the thyroid level is low (hypothyroidism), symptoms such as fatigue, unexplained weight gain, water retention, constipation, dry skin, hair loss, feeling cold, or depression may ensue. It is also related to healthy testosterone levels, bone density, sharpness of mental function, and the rate at which we burn calories. The thyroid hormone is often considered the master hormone under the direction of our pituitary gland.

WHAT THIS MEANS FOR YOU

In wellness healthcare—as opposed to the "sickcare" to which most people are accustomed—it is important to get yourself checked out by an endocrinologist or other physician specializing in HRT to test your hormones. This preventive testing can determine if you are experiencing a hormonal imbalance. As with all the other information in this book, or any book about health, you simply cannot go it alone. You need professionals in your corner who will test you and give you baseline results from which to start. Each individual body is different. Hormone replacement without correct interval blood testing is negligent.

> You need professionals in your corner who will test you and give you baseline results from which to start. Each individual body is different.

DHEA AND LONGEVITY

DHEA is a steroid hormone that is produced by the adrenal glands, and secondarily the gonads and the brain. It is the most abundant circulating steroid in humans and is known to increase in production with regular exercise. It is a precursor to testosterone and the estrogens. Interestingly, the "longer life expectancy" theory brought about by calorie restriction is associated to increased production of DHEA. Athletes in the Olympics and other major sports are banned from this steroidal hormone because of its performance enhancement.

HGH, human growth hormone, is said to slow aging. This hormone is produced by the pituitary gland and is the jet fuel of childhood growth and maintains tissue and organs throughout life. Growth hormone deficiency in adults is rare and may be caused by a tumor on the pituitary gland. Injections, by prescription only, are given for treatment. But what about healthy adults? What have studies proven? The information available is limited, but it does appear that HGH injections can increase muscle mass and reduce the amount of body fat in healthy older adults. If you're over 45, you may want to consult with an age management hormone replacement specialist in your area. First, strive for cardiorespiratory fitness and nutritional excellence. Then, if your blood studies show it's necessary, add in **biodentical** hormone replacement therapy.

Balancing out your hormones with supplementation can help you feel and look younger, especially when combined with cardiorespiratory fitness and nutritional excellence.

Ultimate Health VIPs

1. Our hormones work in concert with physical fitness, good nutrition, proper sleep, and stress reduction/spiritual wellness to produce a symphony of Ultimate Health.

2. Hormones are messengers of the body.

3. Most people begin losing optimal production of many hormones at or around age 30 and fail to take action to adjust, thereby preventing their body from operating at peak performance.

4. Testosterone is an example of an important hormone. Low testosterone could be behind a lethargic sex drive, brain fog, and lower metabolism.

5. Doing annual blood labs and studying your hormone levels with your health team to ensure optimal ranges can have magnificent results on your body's functioning and aging.

6. Taking care of your hormones is important for everyone—not just for women during menopause.

7. Low thyroid levels are frequently the cause of persistent fatigue, constant coldness, and female hair loss, and may contribute to depression.

CHAPTER 12

VITAMINS

Vitamins help your body function optimally. Are you getting your blood tested regularly so you know what supplements you need?

Vitamins and nutrients are important for a strong, healthy body, and the best way to get them is from natural food sources. Supplements are available when that's not possible, and your physician can tell you what you need to take on a daily basis after testing your blood.

Some people are as disciplined about taking their daily regimen of vitamins as they are about brushing their teeth and getting dressed. It is just a normal part of their routine. Others fail to see the need, take supplements sporadically, or ignore them altogether. Recent research is more and more convincing that vitamins and nutrients really do matter.

Fast Facts

- The ideal multivitamin is a whole-foods product loaded with antioxidants and powerful minerals.
- Obtaining vitamins from food (blueberries, avocados, bananas) is the purest source.
- Vitamins such as vitamin C are powerful antioxidants that help fight against cancer.
- Vitamin B gives you energy that can help you to think and perform better.

Your Real Age

Vitamins and nutrients can help you look and feel much younger than your actual chronological age. On top of that, vitamins can help ensure you are getting the nutrition your body needs to operate properly, grow muscle, think clearly, and live in ultimate health.

Vitamins and nutrients can help you look and feel much younger than your actual chronological age—especially if you are determined to be deficient.

A vitamin is a simple organic compound required as a vital nutrient in tiny amounts by an organism. As an organic chemical compound is technically called a vitamin when it cannot be synthesized by our bodies and must be obtained from our diet. There are 13 essential vitamins. *Essential* simply means that they must be obtained from outside sources in order for the body to work properly.

The first step on the path to understanding what you need is to get a medical team member to test your blood in order to determine your levels. By working with a physician, endocrinologist, and/or a nutritionist to direct your own dietary therapy, you will have a good starting point and baseline from which to make decisions. Once you know how to supplement in a healthy way, you can enjoy more vitality and energy—and make smarter choices. Adding a nutritional supplement program to your life (in combination with physical fitness) is perhaps the single fastest solution to positively influencing the effects of aging on your body's cells. Some people use hormone therapy to regulate their bodies, and that, along with the proper nutrition, can determine how your body will heal and thrive in the future.

We can't advocate hormone therapy for you because it's a personal decision, like supplementation and other decisions. Only you and your own medical team know what's best for your body. But you do need the proper vitamins and nutrients, and this book is a wake-up call. Now is the time to get your blood tested.

The two most essential elements of great health are exercise and nutrition. First, get your vitamins and nutrients from your natural food. Second, supplement with vitamins if your medical team feels it's valuable. The essential vitamins are A, D, E, K, and C, along with the Bs. In the B family there are: B1, B2, B3, B5, B6, B7, B9, and B12. (When B vitamins were being discovered, they were assigned names in order by number. The number does not mean anything in particular.) Here's more detail on vitamins:

Vitamin A (Beta Carotene)
Health benefits:
- Can neutralize free radicals
- Protects eye health

Where to get it:
- Oranges
- Ripe yellow fruits
- Leafy vegetables (especially dark green)
- Carrots
- Pumpkin
- Squash
- Spinach
- Liver

B1 (Thiamine)
Health benefits:
- Improves myelin sheath (nerve coverings) development, brain function, energy, memory, and cardiovascular support

- May help reduce symptoms of multiple sclerosis and other disease, like cirrhosis

Where to get it:
- Meat
- Green leaves
- Pork
- Oatmeal
- Brown rice
- Vegetables
- Potatoes
- Liver
- Eggs

B2 (Riboflavin)

Health benefits:
- Cellular function
- Migraine support and relief
- Antioxidants

Where to get it:
- Oranges
- Eggs
- Lean meat
- Milk

Note: Riboflavin is damaged by exposure to light. Foods with riboflavin should not be stored in glass containers that are exposed to light.

B3 (Niacin)

Health benefits:
- Fights high cholesterol, diabetes, cardiovascular disease, and osteoarthritis
- Helps the body make various sex- and stress-related hormones in the adrenal glands and other parts of the body
- Improves circulation

All the B vitamins are water-soluble, meaning that the body does not store them.

You can meet all of your body's needs for B3 through diet. It is rare for anyone in the developed world to have a B3 deficiency unless they are an alcoholic.

Where to get it:

- Eggs
- Dairy
- Beets
- Salmon
- Swordfish
- Tuna
- Anything containing tryptophan

B5 (Pantothenic Acid)

Health benefits:

- Regulates hair growth
- Responsible for hemoglobin production and metabolism of toxins by the liver
- Plays a critical role in cell division
- Crucial for life and growth

Where to find it:

- Eggs, dairy, and most foods

B6

Health benefits:

- Helps break down fats, carbohydrates, and proteins so they can be absorbed more easily
- Essential for red-blood-cell formation, antibody production, and normal brain function
- Cardiovascular benefits

Where to find it:

- Cereal
- Tuna
- Potato
- Chicken breast
- Bananas

- Broccoli
- Sunflower seeds
- Tomato sauce
- Carrots

B7 (Biotin)

Health benefits:
- Promotes hair and nail growth
- Facilitates healthy metabolism

Where to find it:
- Vegetables
- Green plants
- Fruit
- Milk
- Rice bran
- Wholemeal products
- Eggs
- Avocado
- Spinach
- Peanuts
- Cauliflower
- Yeast
- Beef liver

Biotin is found in many foods, but the best sources are beef liver and brewer's yeast. Egg yolks, nuts, and whole grains are also good sources.

B9 (Folic Acid)

Health benefits:
- Facilitates growth and development
- Encourages nerve and brain functioning
- May help reduce blood levels of the amino acid homocysteine (elevated homocysteine levels have been implicated in increased risk of heart disease and stroke)
- May also help protect against cancers of the lung, colon, and cervix
- May help slow memory decline associated with aging

- Critical for pregnant women to prevent birth defects such as spina bifida

Where to get it:

- Dark leafy greens
- Broccoli
- Citrus fruits
- Beans
- Avocado
- Beets
- Celery
- Carrots
- Sunflower seeds
- Dried herbs
- Asparagus

B-complex vitamins are needed for healthy skin, hair, eyes, and liver. They also help the nervous system function properly. All B vitamins help the body to convert food (carbohydrates) into fuel (glucose), which is used to produce energy. These B vitamins, often referred to as B-complex vitamins, also help the body use fats and protein.

B12

Health benefits:

- Brain function
- Formation of blood
- Helps preserve the integrity of the central nervous system
- Helps prevent anemia

Vitamin C

Health benefits:

- Helps fight against cancer and heart disease
- Decreases cholesterol and triglycerides
- Repairs and regenerates tissues
- Aids in the absorption of iron
- Lessens the duration and symptoms of the common cold, especially when taken in combination with 10 mg of zinc

Where to get it:

- Apples
- Asparagus
- Berries
- Broccoli
- Cabbage
- Cauliflower
- Citrus fruits
- Fortified goods
- Kiwi
- Leafy greens
- Melon
- Peppers (especially red bell peppers)
- Potatoes
- Tomatoes

Coenzyme Q10 (CoQ10)

CoQ10 naturally decreases with age and tends to be low in the setting of certain medical conditions such as cardiovascular disease, HIV/AIDS, cancer, Parkinson's disease, and diabetes. Medications such as statin drugs (which are prescribed to lower cholesterol) are known to decrease levels of CoQ10. Supplementing with CoQ10 has been shown to help with muscle pain associated with taking statins. In Europe, it is not uncommon to prescribe a statin drug concurrently with CoQ10 for this very reason.

Health benefits:

Studies suggest that it may help healthy functioning of the heart, treat cardiovascular disease, high blood pressure, congestive heart failure, and heart attack. Some evidence demonstrates that CoQ10 could help slow the progression of Alzheimer's and dementia.

Where to get it:

- Organ meats (heart, liver, and kidney)
- Red meat
- Fish
- Oils from sesame and grape seed

Essential Fatty Acids (Omega-3 and Omega-6s)

Most people are unaware of their Omega 3 vs. 6 levels.

Health benefits:

• Lowers blood pressure

• Helps lower triglycerides (fats in the bloodstream)

• Helps lower low-density lipoproteins (LDL)

• Helps prevent asthma by reducing inflammation in the airways

• Omega 3 helps relieve joint pain and stiffness by decreasing inflammation

• Helps quell chronic gastrointestinal inflammation in cases such as Crohn's disease

• Linked to preventing Alzheimer's disease and depression

Where to get it:

Because humans are unable to make essential fatty acids, we either have to get them from our diet or from supplements. The most beneficial essential fatty acids are the Omega-3 fats found in salmon and other deep-water fish and their oils; walnuts and walnut oil; flaxseeds and flaxseed oil; and legumes. The ideal ratio of Omega 3 to Omega 6 is 1:4. The typical Western diet is 1:10 - 1:30.

Vitamin D

Most people believe vitamin D is a vitamin, but it is actually a crucial hormone. Have your vitamin D level checked. If your vitamin D level is below 30, supplementation is strongly advised. An ideal blood level is in the 40 to 50 range.

Health benefits:

• Normal central nervous system development and function

• Healthy immune system function with suppression of certain cancers

• Bone formation and preservation

• Healthy cardiac function

• Protects against seasonal affective disorder (SAD), a form of depression

Where to get it:

• Sunshine

• Salmon

• Egg yolks

• Cheese

• Beef liver

- Tuna
- Mackerel
- Fortified milk
- Supplements

Vitamin E

Health benefits:

- Helps maintain proper function of cardiac and other muscular tissues
- Assists in the formation of red blood cells
- Has a positive effect on the immune system
- May also aid in preventing heart disease, cancer, diabetes, and symptoms of Alzheimer's

Where to find it:

- Vegetables
- Oils
- Avocados
- Spinach
- Whole grains
- Wheat germ
- Nuts

Vitamin K

Health benefits:

- Essential nutrient necessary for blood clotting
- Helps protect and strengthen bones
- Helps prevent calcification of arteries
- Helps provide protection against liver and prostate cancer

Where to get it:

- Kale
- Spinach
- Leafy greens
- Brussels sprouts
- Parsley
- Broccoli
- Cauliflower

Probiotics

Health benefits:

Probiotics are live microorganisms ("friendly bacteria") that help keep the microflora in the human gut in balance. They help to support the immune system, fight against "bad bacteria," and help the body digest and absorb nutrients. Because a large amount of our immune system resides in the gut, it is very important to support the health of the gut by taking probiotics. Probiotics are especially helpful in the setting of antibiotic therapy or previous antibiotic therapy, diarrhea, irritable bowel syndrome, and urinary tract infections.

Where to get it:

- Yogurt
- Miso
- Tempeh
- Kefir
- Sauerkraut
- Supplements (These should have both a manufacturing and an expiration date on the bottle. Look for a brand that states on the label that it contains live cultures.)

Vitamins are critical to your body functioning properly. To live in Ultimate Health, make sure your blood is tested to determine if you're deficient in any area. If you're low on vitamin D, for instance, the result could be devastating to your overall physical health and wellness in the long term. Vitamin D is an essential nutrient in your body. Other vitamins, such as B, help increase and sustain energy levels and, if you are low, it might result in a diminished energy level and ability to think and concentrate.

Over-supplementation is just as bad as under-supplementation, and some doctors don't endorse supplementation at all, so it's important to seek a professional to guide you. Know your body, know your numbers, and then take measures to feed your body with the proper nutrition and vitamins and minerals it needs for cellular repair, growth, and overall health.

Ultimate Health VIPs

1. Many vitamins are deficient in people's bodies. At a minimum, a strong, daily multiple vitamin is just good, simple practice.
2. Vitamin C is a powerful antioxidant that helps to fight against cancer and heart disease. Citrus fruits, berries, dark leafy greens, and peppers are natural sources.
3. Vitamin D has huge benefits and can be obtained through sunlight and other sources. Some studies have shown that up to 80 percent of Americans have substantial to very unhealthy low levels of Vitamin D.
4. CoQ10 assists in maintaining good cardiovascular health and may slow the progression of Alzheimer's. Organ meats, fish, sesame, and grape seed oils are all excellent sources.

CHAPTER 13

CALORIC MANAGEMENT

A calorie is a unit of energy. It is a measure of the energy we generate with every task we do, as well as a measure of the energy delivered by a food we eat. How well do you know your body and how you balance what you eat versus what you need to perform? This knowledge allows you to make better daily choices . . . and to live in Ultimate Health.

By understanding how your body processes foods and burns calories, you can be leaner and healthier this year than you were a decade ago. When we embarked on the journey to write this book, we knew that we wanted to include caloric management in a chapter because it really is true that you are what you eat. Many people simply ingest too many calories a day! And others aren't aware of how what we eat impacts the skin, hair, nails, body weight, and internal organs. Managing how much food we ingest each day is an important part of fitness.

Even if you have lived a sedentary life, it's not too late. You can start adopting healthy habits today that will transform your life. Anything is possible.

You can become an athlete, even run a marathon if you want to, lose ten to fifty pounds (or even more!), build lean muscle, and live an active, energetic life!

You can turn back the hands of time by educating yourself, shedding excess pounds, and adopting a disciplined nutritional program.

You can turn back the hands of time by educating yourself, shedding excess pounds, and adopting a disciplined nutritional program.

KNOW YOUR BODY

Educating yourself about the foods and energy you provide your body is a very important step toward Ultimate Health. Not all calories are created equal! Some foods will leave you hungry and tired shortly after eating them, but others provide fuel that will get your mind and body operating more efficiently.

Once you know what to look for on your way around the grocery store, you can surround yourself with healthy options. But first, understand how your body operates. Each one of us is unique. Some people have a slow metabolism and seem to gain weight easily, while others have an overactive thyroid or very high metabolism that burns fat. Which one are you?

METABOLISM

It's important to understand the relationship between metabolism and calories. Your metabolism is the combination of all the molecules, hormones, and other chemical cell messengers that regulate the rate at which you burn calories. As you eat, the enzymes in your digestive system break down the food. It is a complex process where proteins turn into amino acids, and carbohydrates turn into glucose. Fats break down into fatty acids. Hormones play an important role. The blood brings each component to the cells and sets off a chemical reaction that determines how each is used, or metabolized.

Multiple small, balanced (complex carbohydrate, protein, and healthy fat) meals during the day will keep your metabolism running at a steadier rate than a couple of large meals. You tend to feel better when you do not have large peaks and valleys in your blood sugar levels that result from bigger meals or high sugar or carbohydrate sweets or snacks. As part of those small meals or snacks, try to work in some nuts. Breaking down complex foods like nuts, fiber, and peppers (especially spicy ones) have been shown to boost your metabolism and burn more calories. As with anything, eat in moderation.

> Multiple small, balanced (complex carbohydrate, protein, and healthy fat) meals during the day will keep your metabolism running at a steadier rate than a couple of large meals.

How many calories do you need in a day? The answer varies depending on the individual. Overall, caloric restriction is one of the best ways to lose weight and keep it off if you can maintain a lower caloric restriction. The average person uses between 1,500 and 2,000 calories on an average day. When you eat less than that, you burn sugar, protein, or fat stores to make up the difference, and you lose weight. That sounds simple enough—and we have all tried various diets—so why is staying at our ultimate weight and performance level so difficult? Because not all calories are equal some satisfy your body's needs, but others just send signals to your brain to crave more.

CALORIE: A UNIT OF HEAT USED TO EXPRESS THE ENERGY VALUE OF FOOD.

It may seem difficult to understand how food manufacturers arrive at that number you see on the side of the candy wrapper under the word *calo-*

ries. A pound of fat stores about 3,500 calories, and in order to lose a pound of fat, you need to burn an extra 3,500 calories. To lose a pound in one week, that would mean creating a calorie deficit of 500 calories per day with diet, exercise, or both. That is why when we reduce calories and stay sedentary, not much happens. But when we reduce calories and increase our energy expenditure through exercise, we get leaner.

Have you ever been on a diet? Diets can help you lose weight, but then you've got to be committed to a lifestyle change, and healthy habits, to keep it off.

The "Mediterranean Diet" for instance, is not a "diet" for those who live in that region. It is a "Mediterranean Lifestyle" made possible by the foods they are naturally surrounded with, such as olive oil, nuts, fruits, vegetables, and fish, which are high in Omega-3s and low in polyunsaturated fats.

Just a few small changes in your diet, habits, and lifestyle can have a major impact on your metabolism and your body's natural ability to burn fat and build muscle.

CARBOHYDRATES

Definition: Any of a large group of organic compounds occurring in foods and living tissues and including sugars, starch, and cellulose.

One key to controlling your metabolism and hunger is educating yourself about the glycemic index (GI) of the carbohydrates in your diet. The glycemic index ranks carbohydrates from 0 to 100 according to how they raise blood sugar levels. Glucose has a glycemic index of 100. When you eat pure sugars, your blood sugar rises and then crashes, leaving you tired and craving more food. Have you ever experienced that feeling after eating a candy bar, donut, or chips? You want more soon after you are done. Foods like white rice, potatoes, and other carbohydrates have a glycemic index as high as table sugar.

Foods with a low glycemic index (55 or less) include fruits and vegetables, beans, nuts, and whole grains. Medium levels (56-69) are found in sweet and baked potatoes, whole wheat products, and brown rice. High levels are found in white bread, white rice, most processed cereals, and foods with added glucose. Foods with a high GI are rapidly digested and result in large increases in blood sugar. They also tend to cause a rapid decline in blood sugar, which leads to fatigue after eating them. Foods with a low GI are digested more slowly and cause a more gradual rise in blood sugar and insulin release. These have proven to decrease weight gain, improve performance, and lower the risk of diabetes and heart disease.

Studies have shown that the higher the GI of the foods eaten for breakfast, the higher the calories people eat for lunch. We stressed earlier the importance of eating breakfast; now we are stressing that what you eat will set the tone for your hunger throughout the day.

As blood sugar levels increase, insulin is released in response. Insulin is an important factor in your metabolism and originates in the pancreas. Perched behind your stomach, the pancreas plays a critical role in how the body reacts to food. Maintaining low levels of insulin allows your body to more easily tap into your stored fat for fuel. If there are high amounts of insulin in your blood, your body does not tap into your fat stores for fuel.

The real takeaway message concerning carbohydrates is to choose those that have a low glycemic index and are high in fiber.

COMBINATIONS FOR ULTIMATE HEALTH

If you can manage it, try to add a healthy protein to every meal. This combination will give you hours of energy and is great at curbing your appetite. Be aware that just eating low-fat foods or watching calories can easily lead to insulin resistance and weight gain if you're not also aware of the glycemic index and hidden sugars in carbohydrates.

Combining low glycemic, high-quality foods, such as leafy greens and colorful fruits and vegetables with lean proteins, is the best choice for Ultimate Health. The body burns more calories digesting protein than it does burning the calories in fat or carbohydrates. Healthy sources of protein include organic white meat chicken, fish, turkey, organic lean beef, nuts, yogurt, tofu, beans, eggs, and dairy.

> We have to be aware that just eating low-fat foods or watching our calories can easily lead to insulin resistance and weight gain if we are not also aware of the glycemic index and hidden sugars in carbohydrates.

STRATEGIES FOR SUCCESS

We have all had times when we vowed to start eating healthier and take better care of our bodies. "Eating healthier" sounds easy enough; why, then, is it so difficult to actually begin and maintain the healthy diet and lifestyle we desire?

Many of the popular diets are far too restrictive, while others are confusing and offer too many contradictions. Eating just carbohydrates or especially high fat and protein or all liquid might work well for short-term weight loss, but the odds of achieving lasting success with such drastic measures are very low.

Another obstacle to long-term success is the surprising amount of sugar and salt hidden in the processed foods throughout our grocery aisles. To some extent, decreasing sugar and salt in your diet is like quitting smoking. Your body craves it and may not feel satisfied without it. Because of the way foods have been produced, it is not uncommon for the body to crave the added sugar or salt in many foods. In some respects, this can be an even harder addiction to address than cigarette smoking because the cause of the addiction is so well hidden in our foods. It can take considerable effort to tell which foods are healthy and low in sugar and which ones are packed with sugar and calories. "Fat-free" items may seem like a great choice, but they may have so much sugar in them that they are actually counter-productive for your diet. Soups or seasoned rice would also seem like excellent choices, but they may have shocking amounts of added salt. Reading labels really helps guide you to understand what foods contain excess sugar and salt so that you don't buy them in the first place.

> The most important advice in caloric management is to exercise, exercise, exercise! Most people, if they are really honest with themselves, do not move their bodies nearly enough.

DON'T SET LIMITS

No matter how old you are or what your fitness level is, it's not too late to start. Jack Lalane was 90, but remained committed to a healthy life each day, and even in his ninth decade he had a daily exercise routine more vigorous than most thirty-year-olds! Sure, you could say he is the exception in a society where obesity has risen to epic proportions. But with dedication, discipline, and commitment, his level of fitness is possible. A slim, strong, muscular body is possible, no matter how old you are. How healthy do you want to be? After reading this chapter, ask yourself:

- Do I exercise as much as I should?
- Am I eating the right combination of healthy foods?

You have the power to transform yourself from the inside out. Start the journey to Ultimate Health today.

Ultimate Health VIPs

1. By understanding how your body processes foods and burns calories, you can become slimmer, trimmer, and fitter this year than you were a decade ago.

2. Educating yourself about the foods and energy you provide your body is a very important step toward Ultimate Health. Not all calories are created equal!

3. Overall, caloric restriction is one of the best ways to lose weight and keep it off if you can maintain a lower caloric restriction. The average person uses between 1,500 and 2,000 calories on an average day. A pound of fat stores about 3,500 calories, and in order to lose a pound of fat, you need to burn an extra 3,500 calories. To lose a pound in one week, that would mean creating a calorie deficit of 500 calories per day with diet, exercise, or both. That is why when we reduce calories and stay sedentary, not much happens. Not all calories are created equal. Some help your body strive while others leave you craving more. Take care in the foods you choose.

4. One key to controlling your metabolism and hunger is educating yourself about the glycemic index (GI) of the carbohydrates in your diet. Foods with a high GI are rapidly digested and result in large increases in blood sugar. They also tend to cause a rapid decline in blood sugar, which leads to fatigue after eating them. Foods with a low GI are digested more slowly and cause a more gradual rise in blood sugar and insulin release. These have proven to decrease weight gain and improve performance. Maintaining low levels of insulin is important to allow your body to tap into stored fat for fuel.

5. Knowledge can enhance your life. Read labels to increase your awareness of excess sugar and salt in many processed foods.

Chapter 14
Ear, Nose, and Throat

Preventive testing is as important for the ear, nose, and throat as it is for the rest of your body. It's important to protect your hearing and ear canal from foreign objects and loud noises, to check for cancers, and to maintain good hygiene. Are you getting checked regularly?

The chapter you're about to read contains information on one of the most important aspects of health. Most people pay attention to pains in their bodies and get annual checkups, but oftentimes the ear, nose, and throat are ignored when it comes to prevention. Here are a few common myths:

1. It is not really important to protect our hearing from loud noises such as music through headsets, concerts, lawn mowers, engines, or other environmental noise.

2. Pinching the nose and attempting to blow out with a closed mouth can rupture your eardrums.

3. Smokeless tobacco is not addictive or in any way injurious to oral tissues.

4. A runny nose with sneezing, and difficulty with nasal breathing, is sinusitis.

5. I should not be concerned about ringing in my ears.

PROTECTING THE SENSE OF HEARING

While most of us certainly appreciate the ability to hear music, language, and environmental sounds, ENT specialist, David Price, MD, asserts that the majority of us do not protect our ears from noise damage very well.

Hearing-destructive high levels of noise occurs in our day to day environment through loud music, common machinery (saws, hammers, drills, lawn mowers, loud vehicles, etc.), concerts, auto racing, and gunfire among others.

The noise-rating system devised to help us protect our hearing is rated in decibels (db). This is similar to the Richter scale for earthquakes, where a 7.0 earthquake is not 10 times more powerful, but 100 times more powerful, than a 6.0 earthquake. Your ears can tolerate 85 db of noise for 8 hours before real injury ensues, but only four hours of 90 db noise prior to onset of inner ear damage. At 100 db, we should not have greater than one continuous hour of exposure, and we should not be exposed to greater than 110 db noise if at all possible.

For example, no one should be exposed to racetrack noise levels without quality hearing protection. Earplugs can attenuate noise by 27-29 decibels, but more serious earmuff protection is required for louder scenes. For racetrack exposure, or gun-firing noise, it's important to consider using peltor headphones for adequate noise suppression. Tactical dynamic earphones are available for those quickly moving back and forth from loud noise environments to standard sound levels.

Another area people tend to be unaware of is the effect of certain medications on hearing loss. If you are hospitalized for a serious infection, intravenous antibiotics (streptomycin, amikacin, tobramycin, vancomycin, gentamycin) may need to be administered. This could lead to significant hearing loss from inner ear damage if your physician is not carefully monitoring the antibiotic levels in your bloodstream. This is especially common with gentamycin, which may cause both loss of hearing and loss of balance. These are viewed as serious adverse events and are often irreversible. Let your physicians and nurses know that you are aware of these risks and that you wish to protect your hearing.

Other issues related to the inner ear are problems that produce dizziness, such as infections, vertigo, tumors, and Meniere's disease. Dizziness from the first two is often self-limited and brief, while Meniere's could pose a longer-term problem. All of these issues require the skilled attention of a board-certified ENT physician in order to accurately diagnose and treat the cause.

Vertigo is best described as the experience of dizziness, possibly nausea, and a sense that the room is spinning around you. The most common form of vertigo is BPPV (benign paroxysmal positional vertigo), which is caused by otoliths (think sand particle) being dislodged from the inner ear. A simple maneuver (Eply) can reposition these particles and quickly correct the vertigo in many cases. Vertigo with Meniere's disease is more complicated, requires the care of an ENT physician, and demands a true low-sodium diet. Symptoms defining Meniere's are vertigo, fluctuating hearing loss, and ringing/roaring in the ears. Some people experience tinnitus, which is a ringing or buzzing in the ears or perception of unusual sounds. There are many causes: elevated high blood pressure, overdosing of aspirin, ear canal obstruction, pierced eardrum, middle ear inflammation, inner ear disease and, rarely, tumors. Seek the evaluation of your ENT physician to protect your hearing health.

Doctors perform the first hearing tests on babies at birth, and it's also a good idea to test again before a child starts school. Impaired hearing, just like impaired vision, may contribute to poor school performance and behavioral issues as time goes on. Children are not usually able to properly respond to standard audiometry testing before about five years of age. Your ENT specialist can use special procedures at earlier ages to determine hearing competence.

The Nose

Common problems with the nose include nosebleeds, nasal stuffiness, and foreign bodies. Stuffiness is most commonly positional or allergic in nature and is *not sinusitis*. Sinusitis is defined by facial pain, by pain in the upper teeth, and is often a sinus blockage problem, which may be associated with decreased ease of nasal breathing. Sneezing, runny nose, and blocked breathing are *not* sinusitis but rather rhinitis, typically of allergic origin. Treatment of the stuffy nose often includes the use of antihistamines taken orally or administered by spray. Avoid chronic use of vasoconstrictor sprays such as Afrin as a rebound problem may develop.

Positional (lying flat) closure of the nose occurs when swelling of structures on the down side of the nose close the nasal passages. It might sound simple, but an easy way to reduce stuffiness, in many situations, is to raise the head of the bed with four-inch blocks. The entire body must be elevated with this technique. Attempting to deal with this problem using pillows only almost always fails, as it does not deal with the physics and physiology of nasal blockage and subsequent stuffiness.

Difficult nasal breathing may also result from a deviated nasal septum, which can easily be evaluated and treated by your ENT specialist.

Oral Conditions

Chronic infection of the tonsils may imply a Strep bacteria, and you might need antibiotics. Life-threatening cancers of the tonsils and tongue can occur with chronic abuse of smoking and smokeless tobacco products, so pay attention to your body and also your habits!

While sore throats are often viral in nature and do not require antibiotics, failure to test and rule out Strep bacteria infection may have serious consequences. Rheumatic fever from Strep infection causes heart valve, kidney, and joint trauma, which are typically irreversible.

Voice box (Larynx)

Chronic laryngitis should be taken seriously because it can represent vocal cord abuse from smoking, repetitive screaming or yelling, acid reflux, or something else. Acid reflux effects on the larynx may best be treated/avoided by elevating the head of the bed with four-inch blocks, thereby stopping the acid reflux into the larynx. Using pillows will not work, as the whole body needs to be on an incline to decrease the reflux. All of these are obviously suggestions. In the end, it's important to be your own advocate.

Ultimate Health VIPs

1. Preventive testing is important for the ear, nose, and throat, as well as for the rest of your body.
2. Foreign substance in the ear or nose should be treated by the proper medical expert.
3. It is important to protect your hearing and ear canal from foreign objects and loud noises.

Chapter 15

Nutrition

Food provides nutritional support for your body. It consists of carbohy-drates, fats, proteins, vitamins, and minerals and provides essential nutrients. Are you eating throughout the day to promote good metabolism? Ask your-self: Do you eat slowly and chew well in order to promote good digestion? Do you make healthy choices such as limiting the fried, processed, and high-sugar foods you eat?

You are what you eat.

And that's good news!

You've heard it before—and it's true. The food you fuel your body with determines if you are fit or fat. The choices you make at the breakfast, lunch, and dinner table, and all throughout the day, determine how healthy and strong you will be, how long you live, and the quality of life you'll experience.

Food Is Medicine

You can make positive choices each day starting today that will increase your circulation, reduce blood pressure, and give you a leaner, stronger body. You can choose specific foods to build muscle and sculpt your abs and arms into the frame of a bodybuilder, and you can choose green leafy vegetables and berries that will reduce cardiovascular disease and inflammation.

We all need nutrition; it comes from the food we eat. How aware are you about the food you eat, when you should eat it, how to best combine it, and even what kinds to have around you? It all matters.

The Basics

There are four basic types of cravings: protein, sugar, carbohydrates and salt. And because we are built with these internal cravings, we want to show you in this chapter why digestion, timing, and planning are all critical to making healthy food choices. The problem with cravings is that your body does not always need what you are craving. Good nutrition involves being able to resist certain things that are bad for you and, instead, choose the things that are good for you.

> There are four basics types of cravings: protein, sugar, carbohydrates, and salt.

Protein Cravings

Protein can be good for building strong muscles, and it's also necessary for satisfying the body's hunger. If you're craving more protein to get your mind away from food between meals, try nuts with or without raisins. Nuts are loaded with omega-3s (which help fight heart disease, cholesterol levels, cancers, and many other chronic diseases), unsaturated (good) fats (which help lower cholesterol), fiber (which helps prevent colon cancer and diabetes and helps you feel full), vitamin E (helps prevent plaque in your arteries), sterols (lowers cholesterol), and L-arginine (helps arterial blood flow).

Studies have proven that adding 1/4 cup of nuts to your daily diet can lead to a significantly higher amount of weight loss, lower rates of cardiovascular disease, and a high degree of satiety (feeling full, or satisfied). Try to buy organic nuts when you can because conventional nuts can be contaminated with pesticides (especially peanuts). Just watch the amount of salt added and remember to feel good about yourself while you enjoy them.

SUGAR

If you feel a need for sweets, having a square of dark chocolate or a few berries may be a good solution. You can find several different intensities and flavors of chocolate that you like and you can feel good while satisfying your sweet tooth when you don't overindulge. Research isn't conclusive either way, but we do want to point out that while some studies have shown no benefit, others have shown that dark chocolate increases endorphins and has an anti inflammatory effect.

CARBOHYDRATES

Carb cravings are common but can be deadly to your waistline! Some carbohydrates are good for you, but if you are craving carbs consistently, it's important to find a solution in order to prevent munching on potato chips and other junk food. If you feel like you need a substitute for these, there are many excellent options. There are chips made from lentils, sweet potatoes, and other healthy vegetables—all of which are a much healthier option than classic potato chips. Another option is air-popped popcorn, which has no fat, some fiber, and only about 40 calories per serving. Reach for that instead!

SALT

Another common craving is salty food. If you find that you are reaching for the salt more often than not, try to find low sodium substitutes. A lot of salt is added to the processed foods we buy and chances are good that you are already getting too much. Sodium can lead to weight gain (water retention), hypertension as well as a host of other health issues.

DIGESTION

When it comes to food intake, calories are not the only factor to consider. Some foods cause your body to work harder during the digestive process—especially if you have allergies—while others do not. It is important to know what will digest properly in your system, and it is equally important to focus on chewing slowly to allow the body to absorb nutrients more easily. We all need fiber, for instance, but too much can make you bloated and can inhibit digestion. (Fiber intake is excellent; just be sure to consume enough water!)

But there is much more to food than just what you eat. It is just as important to know *when* to eat certain things, what to mix them with, and how much to take in. When it comes to food, as with other things, timing matters.

> It is important to know when to eat certain things,
> what to mix them with, and how much to take in.

TIMING

Timing is everything. Protein within fifteen minutes of a workout promotes muscle support, according to decades of hands-on experience and input from athletes and bodybuilders. Most fitness models use protein supplement shakes post-workout to get the chiseled results you see on the covers of fitness magazines.

(One can find countless conflicting opinions and studies, but that is not what we are all about. We have spent years conducting hands-on research—with some of the best experts in the world—to create this book. Yet we still do not claim to know it all. Do what is best for you! Listen to your own physician, fitness professional, nutritionist, endocrinologist, and registered dietitian. Gather a strong team around you!)

If you want to eat pasta, timing should be a factor in how your body metabolizes carbs, as you need more hours during the day for fat burning. Accordingly, you should consider pasta as a lunch choice rather than one for dinner.

The average human body uses between 1,500 and 2,000 calories a day, yet there are many factors that determine how many an individual burns. When you consume fewer calories than you burn, you lose weight. That sounds simple enough, right?

Obesity has just passed cigarette smoking as the leading preventable cause of death in America. If it is preventable, why do so many people literally eat themselves to death? Lack of understanding and knowledge plays a big part. Many people understand not to eat sugars and processed foods, yet not many understand why timing is so critical.

The right food at the right time can mean:

• Prevention of diabetes, high blood pressure, and coronary artery disease
• Increased short-term memory accuracy
• Improvement in attention span and decision-making

Most people understand the importance of eating breakfast every day, making the right choices with snacks, balancing proteins and carbohydrates, and reducing heavily processed foods. But actually *doing* the right things takes effort and commitment. Skipping breakfast is associated with a higher BMI and increased obesity risk. If you choose well, studies show you will eat less total calories per day if you eat breakfast then if you skip it.

Whether they feel they are saving time or saving calories, a full quarter of Americans skip breakfast every day. Unfortunately, this is a terrible choice for your body and for your performance in whatever tasks you face on any given day. In several studies, individuals who ate breakfast performed better on alertness and performance tests than individuals who did not. When the individuals switched groups, the test results remained the same.

If you eat just processed carbohydrates or a high-fat diet, your performance increases for about an hour. After that hour, though, alertness decreases and hunger increases! When you eat a high-fiber or a high-protein, low-carbohydrate breakfast, your alertness, concentration, and performance are high for a four-hour period and your hunger often does not return until lunchtime.

> In several studies, individuals who ate breakfast performed better on alertness and performance tests than individuals who did not.

Healthy Snacks

After a good, strategic breakfast, making healthy choices needs to continue throughout the day. Your body craves the added sugar or salt in many foods and may not feel satisfied without it. Instead of waiting for the temptation to hit, keep healthy snacks on hand such as almonds, apples, bananas, berries, celery, other vegetables, or granola and fruit bars.

Get smart and learn to tell which foods are healthy and low in sugar and which ones are packed with sugar and calories. "Fat-free" items may seem like a great choice, but they may have so much sugar or artificial sweeteners in them that they are actually counter-productive for your diet. Soups or seasoned rice would also seem like excellent choices, but they may have shocking amounts of added salt.

One way to really improve your health is through improved snacking. While eating breakfast and eating more fiber and protein during meals will prevent much of the craving for snacks, some snacks can still be a great part of a healthy diet. Tony lost 30 pounds due in large part to changing his food choices and keeping healthy snacks on hand. Snack bags filled with nuts, such as almonds, or cut-up vegetables, like celery or carrots, can be carried with you or kept in your desk—and you can actually feel good about snacking. You want a healthy balance of protein, fat, and carbohydrates for your snacks to achieve the maximal satiety. Again, it is not just *when* or *what* you eat, but also *how* it all mixes together in your digestive system.

If you do not balance some protein in with your snack even if it's a healthy option like fruit, you will likely be left feeling unsatisfied and craving more snacks. Even the healthier sugars in fruit will leave you craving more food when eaten alone. Adding some nuts or other proteins, however, is very good for your health and leaves your brain *and* stomach feeling satisfied.

> While eating breakfast and eating more fiber and protein during meals will prevent much of the craving for snacks, some snacks can still be a great part of a healthy diet.

Eating breakfast, avoiding sugars, and choosing healthy snacks are vital to optimizing your health. Once you make those lifestyle choices, the rest of your diet will fall in line. For lunch and dinner, keep it as fresh and balanced as possible. Most fish is perfect, but lean beef is good as long as you keep the portions small and avoid meats with added hormones whenever possible. You can never eat too many vegetables! Beans are a great source of fiber, nutrients, and protein.

You can educate yourself and enjoy your food even more. Eating a donut may taste great for a minute, but it is rarely worth the increased likelihood of headaches and poor performance for several hours. Instead, enjoy some coffee and oatmeal (or quinoa) with berries, and be proud of yourself as you strive toward your Ultimate Health!

READING FOOD LABELS

One of the most important things you can do to become an educated consumer is to learn how to read food labels. The items that are first on the ingredient list are contained in higher quantities in the product. For example, if sugar is first ingredient on the list, then the product probably has too much sugar. It is a good rule of thumb to limit the sugar grams per serving to less than 10 gm if possible. High-fructose corn syrup (HFCS) is an especially harmful sweetener because it can lead to food cravings, insulin resistance and potentially diabetes. HFCS can be found in foods that may seem "healthy" such as yogurt, granola bars, cereal, and bread as well as soft drinks. Be sure to read the labels and choose a product that does not contain HFCS. Another thing to look for on labels and avoid are trans fats.

Trans fats come from partially hydrogenated and hydrogenated oils found in margarine, shortening, and many baked goods such as cookies and crackers. Trans fats have been shown to contribute to heart disease and nervous system disorders.

The Dietary Guidelines for Americans that came out in 2010 "recommend limiting sodium to less than 2,300 mg a day – or 1,500 mg if you're age 51 or older, or if you are black, or if you have high blood pressure, diabetes or chronic kidney disease." Please keep in mind that the average American typically gets about 3,400 mg of sodium a day. It is very important to read labels on canned and processed foods because they tend to contain large amounts of sodium.

To keep it simple, try to avoid products that have long ingredient lists with more than two words you cannot pronounce. Ideally choose foods that don't have labels such as fruit, vegetables and lean protein. Try to limit your daily intake of sugar, high fructose corn syrup, trans fats, and sodium as a crucial step toward Ultimate Health.

Ultimate Health VIPs

1. Food is medicine. Eat healthily at meals—and consistently every few hours throughout the day.
2. Fresh, organic berries and colorful vegetables are a great choice whether at home or dining out. They contain potent antioxidants that help prevent cancer by fighting free radicals.
3. Avoid sugars and simple carbohydrates. They are burned quickly and can lead to increased cravings.

Exercise: What foods will you eliminate? Make the committment today.

1.

2.

3.

4.

5.

Love your life; live today with gratitude, and joy.

—Tony Jeary

Chapter 16
Skin Health

Your skin is your body's largest organ. It acts as a protective barrier and can even provide clues about the condition of your body internally.

Are you protecting your skin as you should from harmful ultraviolet rays and from environmental chemicals? Do you schedule regular interval full-body skin examinations for skin cancers and skin changes indicative of internal disease in order to ensure your Ultimate Health?

As the body's largest organ, our skin plays several key health roles. Among other functions, our skin protects against infections, maintains our hydration, helps regulate body temperature, synthesizes hormones, and enables production of vitamin D.

Your skin visually depicts your relative chronological age. While genes do somewhat affect the way our skin looks, we can take important steps to look younger and support healthy skin functions through our daily routine of protective habits. When we protect our skin with sunscreen, good nutrition, proper hydration, and avoiding smoking, we slow the destructive forces that lead to sagging and lusterless, wrinkled skin.

The most important steps you can take to look younger and protect the health of your skin are found in your daily skin care routines.

First, here are a few myths:

Myth #1: The highest-number sunscreen provides the best protection.

Myth #2: The best way to get the Vitamin D we need is by sun exposure.

Myth #3: Our nutrition has little impact on our skin health and function.

Myth #4: Changes in the size, color, and shape of moles don't really matter.

Myth #5: Tanning beds are safer than sun exposure.

Myth #6: Not much can be done to slow or correct aging of the skin.

Start thinking about your skin knowledge base. Understanding your skin and the vital role it plays in your life is a key part of your Ultimate Health. Are there deficits in your skin IQ that may be dangerous to your health? What changes in your daily skin care routine could protect you the best?

Were you surprised about any of the myths above? Many people are surprised about Myth #6 and simply accept the aging skin changes in the mirror. But the truth is that there are positive steps you can take to slow, reduce, or even reverse much of the aged appearance of your skin. *Prevention of sun damage is the first, best defense.* Avoidance of smoking and excessive dietary refined carbohydrates (sugar, flour, corn syrup) and controlling or correction of diabetes are key additional factors in your top lines of defense for your skin.

SKIN CANCER—THE MOST COMMON CANCER

Skin cancer is the most common of all human cancers. One in five of us will develop skin cancer in our lifetime. In the United States, more than 3.5

million skin cancers are diagnosed annually. One person dies from malignant melanoma (black mole) skin cancer every hour. There is an epidemic increase in the number of non-melanoma (basal cell and squamous cell) cancers which have increased by 77 percent since 1992.

Ninety percent of non-melanoma and 65 percent of melanoma cancers are attributed to UV radiation from sun exposure. Tanning beds emit deeply penetrating UVA rays and have now been directly linked to melanoma cancer.

With the incidence of skin cancer continuing to rise dramatically, it is imperative to protect your skin well with sunscreen and to have an annual head-to-toe examination with your dermatologist. It might save your life.

TANNING BED DANGER

People who use UV tanners are 74 percent more likely to develop malignant melanoma than those who have never tanned indoors. Given the heavy use of tanning beds today by people between 15 and 30 years of age, we cannot ignore the fact that melanoma is the second-most common cancer for that age range. Not coincidentally, 71 percent of tanning salon customers are females aged 16-29.

The indoor tanning industry has an estimated annual revenue of $5 billion. The international Agency for Research on Cancer ranks UV tanning devices in its Group 1 list of the most dangerous cancer-causing devices.

For decades sunscreen has been used primarily to prevent painful burns. However, medical research has now proven that proper use of broad-spectrum, high SPF (30-50) sunscreen actually helps reduce the risk of both melanoma and non-melanoma skin cancers. Consistent sunscreen use also significantly slows the development of age changes such as brown blotches, redness and spider veins, and sagging. Even if your skin is not sun burning, you are exposing yourself to largely irreparable, cumulative sun damage. Reduce your chances of skin cancer and aging changes by protecting your skin at all times. Make adding sunscreen a part of your daily routine in the same way as brushing your teeth.

Plan for all possible sun exposure, including the significant cumulative day-to-day UVA exposure that comes through driving your car. You should carry sunscreen in your car and have it within reach. As a dermatologist, Dr. Rick constantly thinks about protection from the damaging UV rays of the sun. Tammy is a trail runner and in order to get her exercise in, she sometimes takes unexpected, unplanned runs in between meetings in the middle of the day. She can do this because she has her running gear, hat, and sunscreen in her car. Jennifer has clear skin because she's diligent about protecting it.

None of us would ever consider sitting in a tanning bed. Don't do it. Plan for the outdoors, and defend against harmful rays.

What About You?
Are You Prepared?

If you go to lunch with colleagues and they want to sit outdoors, do you have sunscreen? One hour baking in the sun can do a lot of damage. If you are prepared with quality sunscreen, you're ahead of the game. Plan in advance to protect your skin. *Make adding sunscreen a part of your daily routine in the same way as brushing your teeth.*

Sunscreen Guide

Look for a broad-spectrum chemical sunscreen containing avobenzone, which protects, by definition, against both UVB (burning rays of summer) and UVA (year-round daily rays). The best "chemical-free" sunscreens contain micronized zinc oxide, and they provide the broadest protection available. Choose a sunscreen of SPF 30-50 rating. An SPF 40 sunscreen offers approximately 95 percent of the available protection, while an SPF 80 sunscreen offers only an additional 1 percent protection. SPF numbers above 50 are primarily marketing hype.

In the northern latitudes, the spring and summer months (March through October) are the most significant months for the greatest damaging, cumulative UV damage to your skin. The time of day to avoid the worst sun damage can easily be determined by employing the *shadow test*. If your shadow is equal to or shorter than your height, it's important to apply sunscreen. It is also important to consider protection of the scalp with a sun-blocking hat. Don't forget sunscreen on exposed ears and apply a lip balm containing sunscreen too.

Proper application and reapplication of these broad-spectrum sunscreens plays the most important role in protecting your skin. Get serious about protecting your skin from cancer and premature aging changes.

VITAMIN D AND SUN EXPOSURE

Research has shown that up to 80 percent of Americans are Vitamin D deficient. That's an astounding statistic! Doctors now know that D is actually an essential hormone that plays a crucial role in all our body tissues, enabling normal development of the nervous system and support of immunity against certain cancers.

The American Academy of Dermatology encourages a daily regimen of taking Vitamin D orally. You can't count on sun exposure to provide adequate Vitamin D blood levels, and the risk of increasing skin cancer is too high to bask in the sun.

If your Vitamin D level is below 30 based on blood studies, oral supplementation is strongly advised. A more ideal blood level based on current research would be in the 40-50 range. Yet it's astounding that many physicians are still reluctant to advise their patients to take the 2,000 to 4,000 units of Vitamin D per day that is necessary to maintain or increase their Vitamin D to healthy levels.

WHY IS TAKING VITAMIN D SO IMPORTANT?

Vitamin D also plays a key role in the development and maintenance of bone and helps to sustain healthy cardiac function. It's important to note that taking high doses of calcium won't strengthen bones if you have low levels of Vitamin D and are sedentary. You need the combination of Vitamin D, plus calcium, plus resistance exercise to prevent osteoporosis.

Vitamin D can also help in correcting mental conditions such as SAD,

Seasonal Affective Disorder, which is a form of depression in those with low Vitamin D. Sun exposure has varying effects on those that live in different latitudes and have differing skin types, so for that reason, no set sun exposure ritual can be prescribed to produce adequate Vitamin D levels. It's imperative for most of us to take oral Vitamin D to sustain healthy blood levels.

NUTRITION AND SKIN HEALTH

Our skin thrives on excellent nutrition—both topically applied and what we ingest.

Quality nutrition containing powerful antioxidants (e.g. lycopene, lutein, zeaxanthin, Vitamins C and E, etc.) plays a vital role guarding against infection, building the immune system, repairing wounds, and protecting against the adverse effects of sun exposure. The nutrition that is good for our internal organs also benefits our skin.

Vine-ripened, uncooked fresh fruits and vegetables offer great nutrient density and value while providing the antioxidants and other essential nutrients we need. World Health Organization research shows we experience optimal health when we consume a combination of nine to 13 servings of vine-ripened fresh fruits and vegetables daily. That's a hard goal to achieve unless you are committed to juicing your fruits and vegetables in addition to consuming them with your meals.

Check out a whole food fruit and vegetable concentrate called Juice Plus. It's a respected juicing concentrate of more than 15 nutrient-dense and vine-ripened fruits and vegetables backed by medical research—and Dr. Rick's own personal experience of using it for more than ten years.

CHANGES IN NEW GROWTHS AND EXISTING MOLES

With the incidence of skin cancer continuing to rapidly rise, self-examination is crucial. Request annual head-to-toe examination from your dermatologist and look for changes in the size, shape (border irregularity), and color of your moles. Have your dermatologist check any suspicious change to determine if a biopsy is needed.

Ten Years Younger

Up to 90 percent of the visible changes attributed to aging are caused by the sun. Do you want to look and feel younger? Turning back time and achieving a youthful appearance is possible if you make a commitment to actively use sunscreen, eat right, and take advantage of simple corrective treatments and topical skin care products. Your appearance and sun damage can be largely repaired through a combined application of lasers, peels, fillers, and Botox. Hand rejuvenation techniques are now available to improve thin skin, prominent veins, and age spots. Innovative treatment programs often help patients avoid surgery. These advanced techniques combine to reduce ruddiness and wrinkling and rejuvenate the skin's tone, texture, and luster.

Preventive and ongoing maintenance of your skin, hair, and body starts from the inside out. So don't forget the most important youthful modifiers: high SPF (30-50) sunscreens, a topical retinoid, nutritional supplements, moisturizers, good hydration, and antioxidant-rich foods!

Ultimate Health VIPs

1. Sunscreen is needed year-round for protection against harmful rays.
2. Vitamin D can actually come from the sun and may affect moods when deficient. This crucial hormone assists all systems of the body.
3. With proper nutrition, sunscreen, and skin care, you can reduce the effects of aging and increase a youthful glow.
4. Every one to two years, have a dermatologist do a full-body skin screening for early detection of skin-related abnormalities.

Dig Deeper

www.aad.org
www.skincancer.org
www.asds.net
www.tilley.com — for great sun-protective hats
www.sunprecautions.com — for sun-protective clothing
www.juiceplus.com — for high quality fruit and vegetable concentrate

CHAPTER 17

WHAT YOU DRINK MATTERS

Consuming adequate amounts of water is critical to maintaining ultimate health. Do you drink enough water each day? Do you manage your alcohol intake? Do you drink too much soda or other high-sugar drinks?

You may have read a lot of health books over the years, but chances are that you have never read one with an entire chapter devoted to liquids. Today, research proves that what we drink matters to sustain Ultimate Health and keep our organs and skin hydrated. When someone is not properly hydrated, it often shows up in their skin, mood, and energy levels.

The human body is made up of 60-90 percent water. Without adequate hydration by drinking water, your cells can become dehydrated. A lack of water can tax your organs, reduce function, dry out your skin, and lead to serious health complications and even death. Because water is so essential to your longevity and Ultimate Health, we want to help you understand how to adopt habits that will help you stay hydrated and make the right choices when it comes to what you drink. Does your environment include the right liquids?

NOT ALL LIQUIDS ARE CREATED EQUAL!

Chances are in any given day, you have the opportunity to choose soda, water, juices, coffee, tea, wine, beer, or other alcoholic beverages. None of those (in moderation) are bad for you, but any one of those in excess can be damaging to your health.

If you drink juice every day for breakfast, you might think you are making a healthy choice. Yet you are very likely taking in way too many excess calories! Tony used to drink two large glasses of orange juice each day with breakfast until he decided to lose weight and follow the advice of trainers, physicians, and nutritionists. His team advised him to make a better, low-sugar choice, so now he drinks water instead. Only occasionally will he drink juice.

WATCH OUT FOR HIDDEN CALORIES

Few things demonstrate hidden sugars better than the beverage aisle at the grocery store. Perhaps the best place to start your commitment toward Ultimate Health is by avoiding this aisle completely. There are 3,500 calories in a pound, and switching from one soda per day to water could substitute out 15 pounds over the course of a year. Diet soda would seem like a relatively healthy option, but a nine-year study from the University of Texas Health Science Center in San Antonio found that those who drank diet soda had a 70 percent greater increase in waist size over that period than those who drank regular soda or no sodas at all. People that drank two or more diet sodas per day had five times the increase in waist size!

A study in the *American Journal of Clinical Nutrition* found that, in a group of 810 male and female research subjects recruited from multiple states, liquid calorie consumption had a greater impact on weight than solid calorie consumption. Wow. Now that's a revelation for most people.

Another source of highly caloric, addictive drinks is lattes and blended iced coffee drinks. The next time you are at a coffee shop, ask to look at the nutritionals (or do it online). It's amazing how many calories, sugar grams, and fat grams are in those drinks. They can also be addictive and very expensive. It is much better to make your coffee drink at home so that *you* have control and knowledge of what is going into it.

Drinking healthier can add years to your life and regenerate your cells. Eliminate sugary, high-calorie drinks. Watch your liquid intake of diet drinks, alcohol, and even fruit juices.

Start developing healthy drinking habits and watch your waistline shrink. Most people are surprised to discover the true number of calories they are actually consuming.

Here are six easy things you can do:

1. Surround yourself with water.
2. Keep easy and healthy drink options in your car, like the vitamin or flavor packets you can easily put into water.
3. Be careful when drinking calories.
4. Keep a liquid log in your phone, note pad, PDA, or a mobile app to count daily calories. There are a lot of resources out there today.
5. Ditch the diet drinks and artificial sweeteners. But if you must drink a soda, drink diet to save the calories.
6. Occasionally choose green tea instead of coffee.

(If you notice we said "ditch the diet drinks," it is not just because they add excess chemicals to your life. Diet sodas have very little nutritional value, and research shows that they can harm you, not help you.)

Now that we have decided to skip the soda or drink aisle, let's discuss what we *are* going to drink.

Water is great; water naturally flavored with lemons, oranges, cucumbers, or whatever else you get creative with is even better. Green tea is an excellent source of antioxidants and has an appetite-suppressant effect. There are many varieties of black tea, oolong tea, and other herbal teas that are very good if you need more variety, but green tea has the most research supporting the most benefits. Recent research is linking coffee with everything from decreased depression to decreased risk of diabetes and Parkinson's disease. However, coffee should be consumed in moderation.

Today, there are also a variety of waters infused with juice, and there is a nice tomato juice/vegetable drink option that gives you additional antioxidants.

Ultimate Health VIPs

1. Keep your body well hydrated.
2. Beware of the hidden calories in fruit juices and sodas.
3. Often, hunger is mistaken for thirst. One glass of water can make you feel full and help stave off hunger cravings!
4. Carefully manage alcohol intake. When under the influence of alcohol, a person often makes bad eating choices (among others) that can impact health and increase risk.

CHAPTER 18

Managing Your Emotions

You are what you think. Until you think something different. Emotion is a complex psycho-physiological experience of your state of mind as you interact with internal and external influences. How are your mood, temperament, personality, disposition, and motivation? All these elements matter; all impact the way our bodies perform. How do you manage your emotions?

We could not write a health and wellness book without mentioning the core element of a human life. Your emotions reside in your heart and mind and govern everything that you do. A negative, toxic emotion can lead to a bad day and infect every aspect of your life. It can spill over into your work, your personal life, affect your family, colleagues, and can grow so deep and depressive that it impacts the way people see you or the way you view yourself. A positive emotional outlook, on the other hand, can be infectious. Everyone wants to be around positive, happy, joyful, and magnetic people.

Emotions are a core element of humanity, and much is spent focusing on them. There are entire industries built on increasing emotional I.Q. and happiness, self-help, motivation, and overcoming depression. There are psychologists, self-help experts, spiritual teachers, and millions of books and products to help you manage your emotions.

> A negative, toxic emotion can lead to a bad day and then seep into everything you do. A positive emotional outlook, on the other hand, can be infectious.

When someone can't control their emotions, or are self-medicating and covering up their sadness, stress, or unhappiness with alcohol or drugs, they're trying to solve an internal problem with an external product. The consequence is a short-term fix. It might make you feel numb, but eventually it wears off. The thing that promised the solution offers more of a problem.

As a doctor, nutritional expert, and personal strategist to thousands, we all believe that emotions are manageable—as long as you make a specific plan that fits your life. Your overall physical and mental wellness, life balance, spirituality, hormones, nutrition, blood sugar levels, belief systems, and psychological outlook have an impact on your emotions. Combine that with your DNA, family history, experiences, life-changing moments, substances you fill your body with, and images you fill your mind with, and it can be an emotional cocktail! There are so many variables when it comes to emotions; it is no wonder they are often in flux.

> Your overall physical and mental wellness, life balance, spirituality, hormones, nutrition, blood sugar levels, belief systems, and psychological outlook have an impact on your emotions.

Each one of us has different strategies for managing our emotions. For

Tony, a large part of maintaining a positive outlook is managing his environment, his workspace, and the things that he looks at and listens to. He puts a lot of planning into framing accomplishments, photos, and significant letters from friends, clients, and family, and has reminders of love and success all around. If you go into his studio, you will see letters from clients, but also a letter from his daughter and photos of significant business endeavors. All of these positive images contribute to a healthy emotional outlook. For others, managing emotions involves taking time away to travel, or participate in a sport or hobby.

What is it that makes you happy?

Ultimately, emotional health is about peace.

Philippians 4:6, 7 says, "Do not be anxious about anything, but in every situation, by prayer and petition, with thanksgiving, present your requests to God."

What could be more peaceful than a peace that comes not from money, emotion, or any material or human thing, but a peace from God? Cultivate your spiritual peace by eliminating toxic relationships, surrounding yourself with positive people, places and things, and taking time alone for prayer and meditation. Life is full of challenges but it's also full of joy.

ULTIMATE HEALTH VIPS

1. Managing your emotions is critical to Ultimate Health.
2. Everyone is different. Be intentional about eliminating the things that make you feel negative and increasing the things that make you feel positive!
3. If you are not seeing the world, your job, or your life in a positive light, make changes!
4. Strive to be content. Contentment creates peace.
5. Avoid unnecessary drama.
6. Create a written list of positive self talk and reminders to inspire you when you need a reminder.
7. Focus on gratitude, what are you thankful for?

Chapter 19

Sleep

Sleep suspends the sensory activity of nearly all voluntary muscles. It accentuates the growth and rejuvenation of the immune, nervous, skeletal, and muscular systems. Are you getting enough sleep? Is it good sleep?

Few things have a greater consistent impact on your daily performance and well-being than a good night's sleep. New research reveals that adequate sleep is directly related to the ability to avoid acute and chronic diseases. Everything from the ability to fight off the common cold to the risk for high blood pressure, coronary arterial disease, diabetes, and chronic inflammation is greatly affected by quality of sleep.

Every individual is different, but for someone who isn't getting enough sleep, behavior modification for greater quality sleep might be needed.

Sleep aids, changing your environment, removing technology, or eating differently during the day might be important factors.

A study at the University of Chicago sleep lab demonstrated the connection between too little sleep, sleep deprivation (SD), and serious health consequences, including critical shifts in key hormones and metabolism along with several chronic diseases, obesity, diabetes, and inflammation.

> Everything from our ability to fight off the common cold to our risk for high blood pressure, coronary arterial disease, diabetes, and chronic inflammation is greatly affected by our quality of sleep.

The kind of sleep you get on a nightly basis directly impacts your health. Sleep deprivation adversely affects metabolism and key related hormones (thyroid, cortisol, insulin, leptin, ghrelin, and others). Sleep-restricted individuals demonstrate reduction in leptin (appetite suppressant) and elevation of ghrelin (appetite stimulant) with subsequent increased hunger for high-carbohydrate (simple sugar) foods. SD has simultaneously become a major factor in the health-challenging abuse of energy drinks and work-related and motor vehicle accidents. *Sleep matters, and sleep deprivation is dangerous.*

If you aren't getting proper sleep it's likely that you are at increased risk of disease and may not be functioning at your optimal level in many aspects of your life. **Snoring might seem harmless, but if someone has sleep apnea, there are extended periods of no breathing, and this can occur night after night for years.** Serious health issues such as hypertension, cancer, and heart disease are linked to sleep apnea, and it's a life-threatening condition that must be corrected with a physician's guidance.

Addressing your amount and quality of sleep is a great starting point toward achieving your goals in performance and long-term health. Every individual body is different. Understand and pay attention to yours, so that you know how much sleep you need. You can then make subtle changes in your diet, exercise programs, and sleeping environment, which can have significant impact on your quality of sleep and thus optimize your energy during the day.

How Much Is Enough?

You can function well on just a few hours of sleep a night as long as you make those nights an exception and not the rule. Sleep matters. And only you will know how your body performs without it. Going to bed with the iPad and the phone and other technology is a bad habit because when you wake up in the night the technology is the first thing you reach for.

Addressing your amount and quality of sleep is a great starting point toward achieving your goals in performance and long-term health. Some sleep experts recommend going to bed by 10:30 PM at the latest in order to be synchronized with your own built-in circadian rhythm (24-hour cycle where brain waves, hormone production, cell regeneration, and other biological activities work towards optimum function). However, others say that the body is individually programmed for different biological rhythms. What is your sleep rhythm?

The Value of Rest

What are you doing to maximize your body's rest and rejuvenation every night? If you find it difficult to fall asleep, or wake up frequently during the night, try to erase all lights and distractive technology from your room. Be intentional about it. What works for you? Maybe it's reading or having a glass of warm milk. Think about your "sleep triggers" and be purposeful about introducing them. Sleep is essential to good health and helps reduce inflammation in the body.

Subtle changes in your diet, exercise program, and sleeping environment can have a significant impact on your quality of sleep and optimize your energy during the day. Eating a meal late at night can result in restless, poor quality sleep. Make the changes until you know what works for you.

Is Your Sleep Environment Soothing?

If you are one of the millions of people who falls asleep watching TV, just stop! Computer monitor light blazing? How about the phone? If any of that is in your bedroom, take it out and concentrate on leaving the activities of the day during the daylight hours. Stop co-mingling daytime activity with nighttime. Your sleep chamber should be quiet, dark, and calm.

One great way to facilitate more sleep is to move more during the day! If you are focused on Ultimate Health, you are already moving your body every day. When you make exercise a priority during the day, your body will crave rest that night. If attempts to come to a natural close of your day with gratifying sleep just do not work for you, consult your physician to do a sleep study or lifestyle analysis.

Getting more sleep should be an intentional part of your healthcare routine. Adopt self-soothing techniques like playing relaxing music and pouring a hot cup of tea, milk, or hot cocoa, or relaxing into a warm bath of lavender oil or bath salts. Work on emptying your mind, and eliminate television if you have become reliant on it to fall asleep. How many times have you had to wake up to turn the TV off?

Most experts advise eating dinner at least three hours prior to bedtime to prevent it from keeping you awake. Every individual body is different; that is why it is so important to use common sense and listen to your body. Some people, for instance, operate just fine on late meals, such as the multitude of thin Europeans who traditionally do not even eat until after nine. That is their normal dinner hour, yet Europeans are far less obese, statistically, than Americans. Ultimately, the point is this: have a great physician on your team and get regular consultations to determine what works best for you.

Getting more sleep should be an intentional part of your healthcare routine.

Ultimate Health VIPs

1. Be intentional about getting more sleep.
2. Diets (calorie restricted) for weight loss are much more likely to fail with chronic sleep loss.
3. Limit alcohol, caffeine, and heavy meals late in the day.
4. Utilize natural solutions that encourage sleep: quieting the mind, exercise, melatonin, a warm bath, soothing scents, music.
5. Start viewing sleep as a tool to elevate your lifestyle and give you more energy during the day.
6. Understand your body, mind, and individual needs.

Chapter 20
Spiritual Wellness

Ultimate Health means maintaining strength in all quadrants—physically, emotionally, intellectually, and spiritually.

Every human life consists of mind, body, and spirit. The spiritual aspect of human life plays a key role in the equilibrium with our physical and emotional characteristics.

Many of us nourish our bodies and cultivate our minds but neglect the spiritual side of our lives. Achieving and maintaining spiritual wellness requires self-assessment, planning, and intentional follow-through.

Your spiritual health also revolves around your worldview, which involves three separate components. Every worldview is summed up in three questions: How did we get here? What has gone wrong? How do I fix it?

Even thousands of years ago, philosophers and teachers wrestled with these questions. Plato, Socrates, Jesus Christ, Einstein, and Freud. In the book of Genesis, an angel appeared to a woman named Hagar and said, "Where are you going? And where have you been?" If you've ever been through a challenging time in your life, you may have contemplated those two questions. Once you can answer those questions, you've got an idea of the plan for your life.

> Ultimate Health requires a system of checks and balances. It rests on a three-legged stool of mental, physical, and spiritual wellness.

Two important elements in spiritual health are *stress* and *margin*. When there is a spiritual deficit we feel stressed, imbalanced, and unwell. We feel a lack of peace. At times of stress, the various venues of our lives suffer, including business, family, and personal health. We perceive the opposite of spiritual health as stress in one form or another.

Physical stress may manifest itself in terms of high blood pressure, sleep disturbances, and weight loss or gain, while emotional stress may result in depression, anxiety, fear, or addictive behaviors.

SPIRITUAL WELLNESS IN
ULTIMATE HEALTH

We are susceptible to greater spiritual imbalance and stress when we place ourselves at the center of the universe. The egocentric worldview is typically manifested by signs of false pride, self-interest, and an attitude of self-sufficiency. This spiritual sickness can be characterized by random desires and impulses, immature selfishness, and an attitude devoid of an understanding of God's will for our lives and our place in the universe. (See Proverbs 3:5, 6; Romans 12:1, 2.)

The American trend of seeking primarily financial wealth, pleasure, personal peace, and avoidance of pain is not a reflection of spiritual wellness. Those are hallmarks of spiritual poverty, and if you're spiritually sick, it's often even worse than being physically sick.

Underneath it all, our lives are ultimately a depiction of what we feed our minds and our spirits. It may be cliché, yet the truth remains: GIGO. Garbage In = Garbage Out.

> We are susceptible to greater spiritual imbalance and stress when we place ourselves at the center of the universe.

How do you react under stress and how do you deal with it? Stress shows up in subtle ways sometimes, though it is often manifested through our daily habits and choices.

When a person exhibits one or more of the following, it can be an indication that it's time to make life changes to reduce stress, increase margin, and strengthen spiritual health:

- Negative reactions
- Constantly impatient
- Addictive behaviors with food, alcohol, drugs, or other escapes
- Explosive temper
- Obesity or weight gain
- Poor quality sleep
- Lack of personal peace
- Escapism from pain
- Disorganization (unusually messy car, house, life)

We can't avoid stress and spiritual challenges in our lives. However, we can take steps to reduce our stress load and strengthen our spiritual health.

Want to know joy and spiritual peace even in the face of life's many stressors? Then we must decide to boldly address the issue of spiritual growth. Stress and our spiritual posture are inextricably linked. Begin by admitting your life also requires "soul" food. With intellectual honesty, willfully assert that there are quintessential elements of human existence that are invisible, beyond human understanding, and outside of our control (greater effort, better education, more meetings, etc.). Even the world's most well known philosophers, scientists, and minds examined the complexity of spiritual growth. Einstein believed in God. Charles Darwin, who believed humans originated from apes, had a history of searching for answers and changing beliefs. He sailed the world, quoting the Bible and marveling about God, and then changed his beliefs later after reading documents by philosophers who were men. But that, in itself, is a wayward plan, because man can't define for you what you're supposed to believe. Your spiritual journey here in this universe is yours alone.

The point is, the ultimate spiritual journey is defined as something you cannot see. You can allow men to influence your beliefs, but if you do you're simply a rudderless ship tossed back and forth in the sea. Spirituality is within you, and it's invisible, the same way that love is. You cannot see love, but you know it's there. You cannot see the spirit world, whether it's your own spirit inside you or the spirit of God, but you know it's there. Some believe that science and spirituality stand opposed, but there are plenty of doctors and scientists who believe in faith and a spiritual connection to the world. You have a mind, body, and soul.

Few would disagree that there's a spirit or soul inside them, yet some just can't wrap their minds around a spirit outside of them (God).

One of life's great enigmas is that we actually gain more control and balance in our lives when we give up the suffering illusion that we can somehow exert ultimate control. And, as Einstein said, the definition of insanity is continuing to do the same thing over and over again while foolishly expecting different results.

> We actually gain more control and balance in our lives when we give up the suffering illusion that we can somehow exert ultimate control. You can be successful and control many things. But sometimes the very best things in life come unexpectedly, from the realm outside of your control.

What are some steps we can take on a daily basis that will profoundly influence growth?

- Take time out before you get out of bed for quiet time each and every day

- Read Scripture: Psalms, Proverbs, John, Romans
- Meditation and quiet reflection—Rom 12:1, 2; Phil 4:6, 7
- Exercise and relaxation techniques
- Prayer—to deepen your relationship with God
- Personal retreat (reflective time alone)
- Journaling—historical road map of your spiritual growth and reflection of God's loving goodness/mercy
- Coaching/accountability partner
- Service to others: discover powerful meaningfulness

Finally, reflecting on spiritual balance and stress, we must address our *overloaded lives*. In his excellent book, *Margin*, Dr. Richard Swenson describes, in piercing terms, how the typical American life is under attack by the disease of *overload*. He defines "margin" as the space that once existed between ourselves and our limits, the reserve with which we meet life's unexpected circumstances and challenges. Whether you're Irish, Japanese, American, British, or Italian, the problem of taking on too much is a universal human issue. Overcommitment leaves people exhausted and without time margin. We are left cut off from time for what matters most and brings meaningful fulfillment. Another aspect of life that minimizes margin time is one's material possessions. The more you own, the more maintenance is required on each thing that you own.

The stuff often actually owns us, requiring our time, energy, and finances.

After reading Dr. Swenson's book, several steps come to mind for gaining margin and relieving the stress that robs our spiritual bank accounts:

- Identify stressors
- Eliminate them from your life
- Guard your heart and mind from additional stressors (Proverbs 4; Philippians 12:1, 2)
- Close the gate, and don't let them in again (read *Boundaries* by Cloud and Townsend)
- Build a strong team for help with life's trials
- Seek God (His Scriptures and His presence) for answers to difficult problems
- Start saying no (set boundaries) and build your *margin*

- Give back—be others-centered
- Be grateful for what you do have

Having and maintaining margin is security, energy, and calm. It is the cure for the disease of overload. Reduce the activity in your life and shift your focus to simplicity doing primarily *High Leverage Activities* (see Tony's book *Strategic Acceleration, Succeed at the Speed of Light*).

Spiritual wellness derives from maintaining margin and boundaries, seeking soul enrichment, and reaching out to give to others.

> Reaching outside ourselves to give to others can alter the lens of our perspective on life while enriching our relationships and making deposits in our spiritual bank.

There is no Ultimate Health, spiritually speaking, without Godly Wisdom. This means seeing things from God's viewpoint and then responding by applying the principles of truth. With this frame of reference we will be able to withstand the onslaught against us in all spheres of our lives. In whatever circumstances we find ourselves, in the most difficult grind of our lives, the preeminence of physical, mental and worldly wisdom gives way and our spiritual reserves are challenged.

Each of use will be mastered by either the physical—the secular, natural worldview — or by the spiritual. At life's end, each one of us is forced to confront the spiritual. What will be the measure of your Spiritual Ultimate Health?

When your spirit, mind, and body are in balance, you live in ultimate health.

Ultimate Health VIPs

1. Spiritual wellness derives from maintaining margin and boundaries, seeking soul enrichment, and reaching out to give to others.
2. The American trend of seeking primarily financial wealth, pleasure, personal peace, and avoidance of pain is not a reflection of spiritual wholeness.
3. Your life is a mix of body, mind, and spirit. If you ignore one aspect, you will feel stress and be out of balance in one or both of the other two.
4. Invest in your spiritual side and nourish your soul by reading and spending time alone in prayer and meditation—every day!

Dig Deeper

- The Holy Bible
- *Margin* by Swenson
- *Boundaries* by Cloud and Townsend
- *The Reason for God* by Keller
- *The Question of God* by Nicholi
- *Forgotten God* by Chan
- *The Relaxation Response* by Herbert Benson

SECTION II -
REFERENCE LISTS OF 25

Lists

25 Healthy Foods

1. **Almonds:** Almonds are the king of the nut family. One serving of almonds (about seven pieces) has more calcium than any other nut, provides you with 15 percent of the daily allowance of Vitamin E, and provides you with plant protein. Almonds are also the only alkaline nut; all other nuts are acid- forming in the body.
   * *These may reduce the risk of heart disease.*

2. **Apples:** "An apple a day keeps the doctors away" sure is a great explanation of what apples do. Apples are very low in calories; 100g of fresh slices contain only 50 calories. Apples are also packed with two very important components, phytonutrients (fights unwanted disease and bacteria) and antioxidants (helps prevent damage to your bodies cells).

3. **Asparagus:** Asparagus is a nutritional powerhouse. It is a good source of vitamin K (important for strong bones and blood clotting) and antioxidants and can help reduce risk of serious health problems like heart disease, diabetes, and cancer.

4. **Blueberries:** Another vitamin-rich fruit that scientists have shown is loaded with phytonutrients that may help prevent chronic diseases, and may also improve short-term memory and promote healthy aging.

5. **Broccoli:** Besides being a good source of folate, broccoli contains phytonutrients. This food is an excellent source of vitamin C and also an excellent source of vitamin A. Broccoli has also been linked to preserving eye health.

6. **Brussels sprouts:** This super food contains a high dose of phytochemicals used in fighting cancer. These "mini cabbages" are also excellent sources of vitamins A, C, E, K, B6, folate, iron, manganese, potassium,

and dietary fiber. Studies have shown that Brussels sprouts, along with other vegetables, actually provide protection deeper than the cellular level to reduce damage of the DNA structure.

7. **Cabbage:** Cabbage contains indoles, which are compounds that significantly reduce risks of breast, colon, and stomach cancer. Cabbage also has the potential to purify your blood and kill viruses and bacterias, and helps to improve your immune system. Red cabbage has an added bonus; the red color contains antioxidants that also help fight cancer.

8. **Cannellini beans:** An excellent source of iron, magnesium, and folate. A single serving of cannellini beans provides more than 20 percent of the recommended daily dose of these nutrients. They are also a good source of protein, providing more than 15 grams per serving.

9. **Eggs:** Eggs are a great source of protein, especially when in need of a break from meats. Eggs are also a highly recommended food, full of vitamins and minerals such as choline and lutein, which is vital for brain function, eye health, pregnancy, and fetal development.

10. **Grapes:** Grapes, green or red, are an excellent source of antioxidants, vitamins A, C, and B6, and folate. Not only do grapes add flavor and texture to a recipe, they also help to prevent heart disease, cancer, and Alzheimer's disease.

11. **Green beans:** Green beans are an important source of both carotenoids, flavonoids, and vitamins C and A, as well as bone-building vitamin K. They are also a very good source of fiber, folate, vitamin B6, magnesium, and potassium. Green beans are rich in iron, niacin, calcium, protein, and omega-3 fatty acids.

12. **Leeks:** Leeks have a positive effect on health and well-being. A leek serving has 11mg of salt. The leek also contains significant levels of manganese (15 percent) and iron (8 percent).

13. **Pears:** Pears have been called "nature's perfect fruit" due to their lack of allergic reactions. One single pear can supply as much as 15 percent of daily vitamin C and copper intake. They are also rich in fiber and supply vitamin A, iron, thiamine, riboflavin, calcium, potassium, and protein. They also contain vitamin E, another important antioxidant.

14. **Peanut butter:** Peanut butter is one of the richest sources of heart-healthy monounsaturated fats. Peanut butter is an excellent source of protein to keep you feeling full for longer, fiber for bowel health, and folate, which can protect against colon cancer and heart disease. In fact, researchers recently reported that a tablespoon of peanut butter five days a week can nearly halve the risk of a heart attack.

15. **Pine nuts:** Pine nuts might be small, but they have significant nutritional value. There are about 11 grams of protein in one half-cup. Pine nuts are also loaded with cancer-fighting antioxidants and pinolenic acid, which is a natural appetite suppressant.

16. **Popcorn:** Who knew the long-loved cinema snack could prevent cancer and help dieters? Popcorn is a whole grain shown to reduce the risk of heart disease and cancer, and just half a small box of popcorn in the cinema is equivalent to one daily portion of brown rice or whole wheat pasta. Popcorn also contains three times more fiber by weight than sunflower seeds, keeping you feeling fuller for longer, as well as balancing your blood sugar levels (so no mood swings or cravings for sweet snacks). Popcorn also helps to lower "bad" LDL cholesterol. It even has a dose of B vitamins to boost your energy levels that keeps you awake longer for your favorite film.

17. **Red beans:** Including small red beans and dark red kidney beans in your diet makes for a good source of iron, phosphorus, and potassium. They are also an excellent low-fat source of protein and dietary fiber. Red beans also contain phytonutrients, helping prevent cancer and disease.

18. **Salmon:** Salmon is a great form of protein. It contains omega-3 fatty acids, a type of fat that makes your blood less likely to form clots that may cause heart attacks. Omega-3s also protect against irregular heartbeats that may cause sudden cardiac death, help decrease triglyceride levels, decrease the growth of artery-clogging plaque, lower blood pressure, and reduce the risk of stroke. In addition to containing omega-3s, salmon is low in saturated fat.

19. **Spinach:** Spinach is high in vitamins A and C as well as folate. It is also a good source of magnesium. Spinach may boost your immune system and can help keep your hair and skin healthy. The carotenoids found in spinach, beta carotene, lutein, and zeaxanthin are also protective against age-related vision diseases such as macular degeneration and night blindness, as well as heart disease and certain cancers.

20. **Sweet potatoes:** The deep orange-yellow color of sweet potatoes tells you that they are high in the antioxidant beta-carotene. Food sources of beta-carotene, which is converted to vitamin A in your body, may help slow the aging process and reduce the risk of some cancers. As well as being an excellent source of vitamins A and C, sweet potatoes are a good source of fiber, vitamin B6, and potassium. And like all vegetables, they are essentially fat-free and relatively low in calories.

21. **Watercress:** In addition to vitamins A and C and beta-carotene, watercress also contains micronutrients that work in tandem with the antioxidants to combat cancer-friendly free radicals in the body. Several scientific studies have linked watercress intake to lowered rates of cancer risk in smokers and nonsmokers alike.

22. **Hummus:** It is a gratifying combination of nutrition when paired with fresh veggies like baby carrots or baked pita chips. Made from chickpeas, hummus is a good source of iron, vitamin C, protein, and fiber. So enjoy the pleasing taste of hummus and skip the cheese dip that can lead to diet sabotage.

23. **Granola:** Look for a granola that contains a variety of nuts and seeds—or make your own, and use as many kinds as you want. Just like oats, nuts are a good way to lower your risk of heart disease. They're high in protein, which gives you long-lasting energy for the day. They're also full of fiber, vitamin E, and selenium.

24. **Sunflower:** These seeds are full of vitamin E, vitamin B1, and minerals and are a great quick snack.

25. **Eggplant:** This is an excellent source of digestion-supportive dietary fiber and bone-building manganese.

25 Unhealthy Foods

1. **Diet sodas:** Take out the sugar and add in carcinogenic artificial sweeteners, combined with the artificial flavors and colors that are in all sodas, and you have a recipe for "Tumor in a Can."

2. **Corn oil:** It has 60 times more omega-6 to omega-3. Omega-6 fatty acids increase inflammation, which boosts your risk of cancer, arthritis, and obesity.

3. **Fat-free salad dressings:** When fat comes out, sugar goes in. Either that or artificial sweeteners. Second, since many of the vitamins in vegetables are fat soluble, taking away the fat from the dressing means fewer of the salad nutrients will be absorbed into your body.

4. **Flavored Coffee Creamers:** Some creamers don't include any actual dairy and are instead made from partially hydrogenated vegetable oil, corn syrup solids, and artificial flavoring. They are also extremely high in sugar.

5. **Yogurt cups with fruit:** These are usually loaded with corn syrup, which doubles the amount of sugar. Tastes great to kids, but sure isn't healthy.

6. **Fruit juice:** There is often more sugar in a glass of fruit juice than in a candy bar or glass of soda.

7. **Processed cheese:** It is high in saturated fat and can be very hard on the digestive system.

8. **Mayonnaise:** It's not so bad if you keep it under a tablespoon or two. But that's just it: most can't keep it to the minimum. You can rack up to 360 calories and 40 grams of fat in a one quarter-cup serving.

9. **Alcoholic beverages:** EMPTY CALORIES!!! The body can't use them as energy, and the liver is forced to break down the alcohol into fatty acids, which then store in the liver. Liver and brain cells actually die with excessive exposure to alcohol.

10. **Processed lunch meat:** It contains lots of sodium. It is also linked to increased risk of colon cancer.

11. **Hot dogs:** Once again, lots of sodium, 520–680 milligrams per 2-ounce serving. Leaner and lower sodium meats are a better option.

12. **Whole milk:** It has an overabundance of fat and cholesterol. Sixteen ounces of whole milk a day adds up to 1,904 calories, 105 grams of fat, and 315 milligrams of cholesterol a week.

13. **Frozen French fries:** One small serving (3 ounces) contains 8 to 11 grams of fat, 390–540 milligrams of sodium, and about 160–190 calories. Plus, due to it being frozen and processed, you are losing most of the nutrition.

14. **Corn-fed beef:** Cows are meant to eat grass. If they are eating grains, it is because the farmers want to beef up their cattle faster in order to make more money. This means a lot less nutrition for us.

15. **Potato chips:** Take out most of the nutrients of a potato and fry what's

left, and that will give you potato chips. They also contain trans-fatty acids that increase your risk of cancer, heart disease, diabetes, and stroke.

16. **Donuts:** Donuts are made from refined flour, white sugar, and oil. They also contain large doses of artificial flavors and colors; that is what makes them look and taste so good. Donuts are lacking in fiber and do not provide you with any nutrients whatsoever.

17. **Sugar-coated commercial breakfast cereals:** Most contain sugar as one of the first ingredients, high fructose corn syrup is usually somewhere on the list of ingredients, and they are made from refined grains. This means that you are getting a load of empty calories first thing in the morning.

18. **Canned soup:** Canned soups that you see lining the shelves of grocery stores tend to be loaded with sodium and trans-fats. You may be able to find healthier options in the health food store, but the best soup is homemade soup.

19. **Bran muffins:** Bran muffins are comprised of two things your body doesn't want in the morning: sugar and refined flour. Both will work to spike your blood sugar, which signals your body to start storing fat, and sets you up for a mid-morning crash.

20. **Chicken caesar salad:** Fatty dressing and parmesan cheese and croutons are what make up a caesar salad. Even a side portion is about 500 calories.

21. **Tuna melt:** Plain tuna out of the can is healthy; tuna doused in mayo, shrouded in melted cheese, and slicked with another layer of dressing is not.

22. **Fruit smoothies:** Many fruit smoothies contain added sugars and high-fructose corn syrup, which means they are actually more milkshake than smoothie.

23. **White bread:** White bread is made from refined white flour. It contains a large proportion of high glycemic index carbohydrates, which contribute to diabetes and the lowering of metabolism.

24. **Bagel with cream cheese:** The bread is bad enough, containing 300 calories and 60 grams of carbohydrates, but tack on the liberal cream cheese schmear and your breakfast is now worse than a Big Mac.

25. **Margarine:** They removed saturated fat from butter and created something worse. Something loaded with trans-fats, a dangerous lipid with more concerning links to heart disease than saturated fat.

25 Terms to Know

1. Calculators

What:

Body Mass Index (BMI): calculated from your weight and height and measures average body fatness. This can serve as a guide to overall health and should be treated as a helpful guide to healthfulness. The BMI measures your height-to-weight ratio to determine your level of healthiness.

Basal Metabolic Rate (BMR): the amount of energy expended by the body when it is at rest in a comfortable position and environment.

Resting Metabolic Rate (RMR): the energy required to perform vital body functions such as respiration and heart rate while the body is at rest. About 50 to 75 percent of one's daily energy expenditure can be attributed to resting metabolic rate.

Why you care:

BMI, BMR, and RMR are all calculators to gauge how healthy you are. These allow you to see where you stand in your health and show you where you might need improvement. Not only can you lose weight working out and eating right, but you can also lose weight by just resting.

What to do:

To know your BMI, BMR, or RMR, you can find calculators online and input your personal statistics, and they will give you your results. However, going to a doctor and having them measured by a professional trained in this area is the best way to make sure you have the most accurate measurements possible.

2. Calories

What:

Calories are units of energy that fuel our bodies. 3,500 calories equals one pound. The actual amount of energy consumed per day is a simple formula: Daily Energy Needed = "Amount your body needs" + "Amount your body needs to do extra things."

Why you care:

Keeping the amount of calories you consume balanced with the amount of calories you burn through regular metabolism and physical activity will keep your weight stable. When you take in more calories than your body burns, your body stores these extra calories as fat and you gain weight.

What to do:

Losing weight requires creating a calorie deficit so that your body burns more calories than you take in. Create this calorie deficit by eating 500 to 1,000 fewer calories than your body needs each day and participating in 30 minutes or more of physical activity on most days of the week.

3. Carbohydrates

What:

Carbohydrates are chemical compounds made up of carbon, hydrogen, and oxygen that join together to form molecules. Simple carbohydrates are single-sugar molecules or two-sugar molecules that have joined together, while complex carbohydrates, otherwise known as starches, are comprised of many sugar molecules, which are all connected.

Why you care:

They provide the body with the fuel it needs for physical activity and for proper organ function. They are an important part of a healthy diet.

What to do:

Choose the best sources of carbohydrates—whole grains, vegetables, fruits, and beans—since they promote good health by delivering vitamins, minerals, fiber, and a host of important phytonutrients. Skip the easily digested refined carbohydrates from refined grains—white bread, white rice, and the like—as well as pastries, sugared sodas, and other highly processed foods, since these may contribute to weight gain, interfere with weight loss, and promote diabetes and heart disease.

4. Cell Rejuvenation

What:

Cell rejuvenation is the regrowth of a damaged or missing organ part from the remaining tissue. As adults, humans can regenerate some organs, such as the liver. If part of the liver is lost by disease or injury, the liver grows back to its original size, though not its original shape. And our skin is constantly being renewed and repaired. Unfortunately, many other human tissues do not regenerate, and a goal in regenerative medicine is to find ways to kick-start tissue regeneration in the body, or to engineer replacement tissues.

Why you care:

The human body is constantly replacing and regenerating cells to maintain proper and efficient function. Different cells—such as blood cells, skin cells, and bone cells—are being replaced at different rates. Fat cells are replaced at the rate of about 10 percent per year in adults. So you could say that, on average, human beings replace all their fat cells about every ten years.

What to do:

Regeneration of cells is a somewhat slow process. To increase your health, it is important to keep a good diet and exercise often. To have Ultimate Health, you need your inside to match your outside. If your body looks good, but you are still unhealthy, that is not where you want—or need—to be. Making sure you take care of your body so that it has healthy cells to build upon is the only way to increase, and maintain, your health.

5. Cholesterol

What:

A waxy, fat-like substance that is found in all cells of the body. Your body needs some cholesterol to make hormones, vitamin D, and substances that help you digest foods. Your body makes all the cholesterol it needs. However, cholesterol also is found in some of the foods you eat.

Low-density lipoproteins (LDL): commonly referred to as "bad cholesterol" due to the link between high LDL levels and cardiovascular disease.

High-density lipoproteins (HDL): seen as "good" lipoproteins since they can remove cholesterol from atheroma within arteries and transport it back to the liver for excretion or re-utilization.

Very-low-density lipoproteins (VLDL): molecules made up of mostly triglycerides, cholesterol, and proteins. VLDLs, also known as the "very bad" cholesterol, carry cholesterol from the liver to organs and tissues in the body.

Why you care:

Cholesterol can be both helpful and harmful to your body. On the good side, it helps build the hormones and cells your body needs. But when you have too much cholesterol, it collects inside the walls of your blood vessels. This can cause heart disease, heart attacks, and strokes.

What to do:

Most of the time, you can take care of your cholesterol by eating right and getting the exercise you need. It is important to eat healthy foods to keep a healthy weight. Check your cholesterol every year or as often as recommended by your healthcare provider.

6. Cortisol

What:

Cortisol, a hormone, is a key player in your body's timeless fight or flight stress response and is vital for supplying energy—fast! Cortisol stimulates the release of glucose, fats, and amino acids into the bloodstream to meet those demands.

Why you care:

Cortisol is essential to life and has many positive effects. It gives the body a burst of needed energy when you are trying to get away from danger; it is an important part of helping your body respond and deal with stress. It also contributes to better memory, increased immunity, and the homeostasis of the body. Cortisol secreted frequently due to chronic stress can lead to unhealthy inflammation in the body. Chronic increased cortisol levels has been linked to increased belly fat.

What to do:

To keep cortisol at healthy levels, reduce belly fat and engage the body's relaxation system. Practice relaxation techniques, increase sleep, exercise regularly, and eat a balanced diet to help lower cortisol levels.

7. Creatine Phosphate

What:

It is an organic compound that provides a quick source of energy for muscle fibers to contract when they need an initial burst of energy. It is found in the brain and provides a burst of energy for neurons.

Why you care:

Cellular development depends upon receiving the proper balance of fresh oxygen, water, nutrients, vitamins and, sometimes, supplementation. Cells rejuvenate with sufficient nutrition, exercise, rest, relaxation, and recreation. It helps you to grow younger on a cellular level.

What to do:

Consume a balanced proportion of healthy foods, including fruits, vegetables, and whole grains. Eat foods that contain an abundant source of iron, calcium, Vitamin K, Vitamin C, Vitamin E, Omega-3 fatty acids, Resveratrol, flavonoids, amino acids, fiber, and enriched antioxidants.

8. DHEA

What:

DHEA is a hormone that is naturally made by the human body. It is used for slowing the aging process, improving thinking skills in older people, and slowing the progress of Alzheimer's disease.

Why you care:

DHEA levels seem to decrease as people get older. DHEA levels also seem to be lower in people with certain conditions like depression. Some researchers think that replacing DHEA with supplements might prevent some diseases and conditions.

What to do:

Consult with a specialist to see if DHEA supplements are right for you.

9. Dietary Fiber

What:

Fiber is the part of plants that cannot be digested. Dietary fiber helps to absorb water and remove waste from the body. Dietary fiber includes substances like cellulose, wax, and lignin—among others. The term "fiber" is actually not the best way to describe it, because many of these substances are not actually fibers. Dietary fiber is grouped as soluble or insoluble. Soluble fiber attracts water and slows down digestion time. Insoluable fiber adds bulk to the stool and helps to prevent constipation.

Why you care:

Fiber, especially that found in whole grain products, is helpful in the treatment and prevention of constipation, hemorrhoids, and diverticulosis. Diverticula are pouches of the intestinal wall that can become inflamed and painful. This inflammatory condition is called diverticulitis. In the past, a low-fiber diet was prescribed for this condition. It is now known that a high-fiber diet gives better results at preventing diverticulosis once the inflammation has subsided.

What to do:

Don't worry about what kind of fiber you are taking in unless you are seeking a specific health benefit, such as eating more soluble fiber to lower cholesterol. Instead, focus on eating a healthy diet rich in fruits, vegetables, whole grains, legumes, nuts, and seeds. This will provide a variety of soluble and insoluble fibers—along with all of the other health benefits.

10. Enzymes

What:

Enzymes are protein-based substances that play an essential role in every function in the human body, including eating, digestion, breathing, kidney and liver function, reproduction, and elimination. In the digestive tract, enzymes break down foods by breaking apart the bonds that hold nutrients together—nutrients that the body will eventually use for energy.

Why you care:

There are several enzymes that the human body lacks, such as cellulase (the enzyme that breaks down cellulose), and phytase, the enzyme that breaks down the phytates and phytic acid we consume in our diet. Because of this deficiency, many people have difficulty breaking down certain foods such as starchy beans, legumes, and nuts. Without the essential enzymes needed for proper digestion, the body may not completely break down those foods to absorb their nutrients. As a result, undigested food in the digestive tract can ferment, causing gas, bloating, and other digestive difficulties.

What to do:

We get more enzymes in our diet by knowing where the most active enzymes are and then eating these foods. Dieting, with an emphasis on raw fruits and vegetables, and complex carbohydrates, as well as supplements, will help put more enzymes in your life. P-A-L Plus Enzymes are among the best-performing enzyme supplement on the market today.

11. Estrogen

What:

Estrogen is a hormone that comprises a group of compounds, including estrone, estradiol, and estriol. It is the main sex hormone in women and is essential to the menstrual cycle. Although estrogen exists in men as well as women, it is found in higher amounts in women, especially those capable of reproducing.

Why you care:

Panic attacks have been linked to decreasing hormone levels in women. Low estrogen levels can cause depression and anxiety in some women. As hormones decrease, the onset of an enzyme called monoamine oxidase (MAO) destroys neurotransmitters. Neurotransmitters that greatly affect mood and emotions are serotonin, dopamine, and norepinephrine. Along with panic attacks, a woman may suffer with low self-esteem, poor memory, and have difficulty concentrating.

What to do:

If you think your estrogen balance is off, consider having your hormone levels checked. Consult with an expert as to whether or not hormone replacment is indicated.

12. Fats:

What:

Fats are nutrients. Fat is crucial for normal body function; without it, we could not live. Not only does fat supply us with energy, it also makes it possible for other nutrients to do their jobs.

Saturated fats: directly raise total and LDL (bad) cholesterol levels. Conventional advice says to avoid them as much as possible. More recently, some have questioned this, as there are different kinds of saturated fats, some of which have at least a neutral effect on cholesterol.

Unsaturated fats: Monounsaturated fats and polyunsaturated fats are two types of unsaturated fatty acids. They are derived from vegetables and plants.

Monounsaturated fats: This type of fat is preferable to other types of fat and can be found in olives, olive oil, nuts, peanut oil, canola oil, and avocados. Some studies have shown that these kinds of fats can actually lower LDL (bad) cholesterol and maintain HDL (good) cholesterol.

Polyunsaturated fats: These are found in safflower, sesame, corn, and cottonseed. This type of fat has also been shown to reduce levels of LDL cholesterol, but too much can also lower your HDL cholesterol.

Visceral fats: a type of body fat that exists in the abdomen and surrounds the internal organs. Everyone has some, especially those who are sedentary, chronically stressed, or who maintain unhealthy diets.

13. Free Radicals

What:

Organic molecules responsible for aging, tissue damage, and possibly some diseases. These molecules are very unstable; therefore they look to bond with other molecules, destroying their health and further continuing the damaging process.

Why you care:

Free radicals are unstable. They do not have an even number of electrons, so they are always searching for an extra electron they can "steal" to become stable. Out in the world, this is a normal process, but in the body, it can result in unnecessary and unwanted damage to healthly molecules of the body.

Free radicals play a key role in several biological processes. They play a part in the work of the white blood cells called phagocytes, which "eat" bacteria and other pathogens in the body. They are also believed to be involved in a process called redox signaling, where they are thought to act as cellular messengers.

What to do:

One way to feed the hungry electron appetite of free radicals is to eat more antioxidants. Antioxidants are molecules often found in fresh foods like vegetables and fruits, particularly in the vitamins found in these foods, including A, E, and beta-carotene. These molecules act like a giant boulder in the path of the snowball, stopping free radicals from causing untold damage. Generally, it is better to get antioxidants from a balanced diet, rather than vitamin supplements, because the body can more easily absorb them.

14. Glucose:

What:

Glucose is a simple sugar that provides the body with its primary source of energy. This type of sugar comes from digesting carbohydrates into a molecule that the body can easily convert to energy. When glucose levels in the bloodstream are not properly regulated, a person can develop a serious condition, such as diabetes.

Why you care:

Glucose is the basic fuel for the cells in the body, and insulin takes the glucose from the blood into the cells. When glucose builds up in the blood instead of going into cells, it can cause problems: the cells of your body become starved for energy and high blood glucose levels may hurt your eyes, kidneys, nerves, or heart over a period of time.

What to do:

Always go for the wholegrain option. Replace white rice with brown rice, and make sure your pasta is whole wheat. Make sure you get as many vegetables into your diet as you can. Be as physically active as possible. It doesn't have to be exercise at the gym; even walking instead of driving, or taking the stairs instead of the elevator, can really help.

15. Glycemic Index

What:

The glycemic index (GI) is a ranking of carbohydrates on a scale from 0 to 100 according to the extent to which they raise blood sugar levels after eating.

Why you care:

Foods with a high GI are those which are rapidly digested and absorbed and result in marked fluctuations in blood sugar levels. Low-GI foods, by virtue of their slow digestion and absorption, produce gradual rises in blood sugar and insulin levels, and have proven benefits for health. Low-GI diets have been shown to improve both glucose and lipid levels in people with diabetes (type 1 and type 2). They have benefits for weight control because they help control appetite and delay hunger. Low-GI diets also reduce insulin levels and insulin resistance.

What to do:

You can purchase books or look online for foods that fit into the glycemic index. Eating foods on this list and avoiding fatty and unhealthy foods is a certain way to make sure you are eating in such a way that you'll stay at a good level of Ultimate Health.

16. Hormone

What:

Hormones are chemicals that carry messages from the organs of your body to your cells. The glands that secrete hormones are part of the endocrine system (pituitary, thyroid, adrenals, and pancreas, to name a few) and work in large part to keep the body's natural balance in check.

Why you care:

Hormones induce, regulate, and control almost all bodily functions. You begin decreasing the production of hormones at age 30. Little by little, your body stops secreting hormones at the same level; therefore, they stop regulating your body, you slow down, and of course, eventually die. The ideal performance range of key hormones can actually make your body seem younger than your chronological age.

What to do:

To avoid health issues as we age, and to repair our bodies more effectively, supplements and even hormone replacement therapy have been made available to keep our bodies feeling and looking young. Have your hormone levels checked by a qualified healthcare professional and take the prescribed regimen toward your ultimate health.

17. Inflammation

What:

Inflammation is the body's first response to an injury or disease. Inflammation informs you that you need to pay attention to an injured or diseased area so that you do not continue to use it and worsen the problem. Your body takes chemicals to the injured area of your body (including white blood cells), and these cells repair and heal the body.

Why you care:

It has been associated with many chronic diseases and even cancer. Your body exists in a delicate place between ups and downs—temps, chemistry, vigilance, and balance of all things. It is called homeostasis. When things get a bit "off" from being "just right," the body has mechanisms to get it back to the middle of where you need it to be. Inflammation is one of those things. Some is good, but too much is potentially harmful—and things can start to go awry!

What to do:

One of the greatest things you can do to fight inflammation in the body is to eat foods that are loaded with antioxidants, compounds that help prevent tissue damage from free radicals.

18. Insulin

What:

Insulin is a hormone that lowers the level of glucose in the blood. It is made by the beta cells of the pancreas and released into the blood when the glucose level goes up, such as after eating. Insulin helps glucose enter the body's cells, where it can be used for energy or stored for future use.

Why you care:

The typical western diet of highly processed, high-glycemic foods—soft drinks, candy bars, bagels—causes blood sugar to rise dramatically, which makes the level of insulin rise, causing blood sugar to plummet. When insulin levels stay elevated this way, the body continuously uses glucose for fuel rather than both glucose and fat. In short, you become a fat-storage factory.

What to do:
Eating small low-glycemic portions at frequent intervals is good for maintaining stable blood sugar. One study showed that eating six small meals daily led to a decrease in overall and LDL ("bad") cholesterol levels.

19. Melatonin

What:
Melatonin is a hormone secreted by the pineal gland in the brain which helps to regulate other hormones and maintains the body's internal clock.

Why you care:
It helps with sleep and improves daytime alertness. Preliminary evidence suggests that it may help strengthen the immune system and possibly help prevent certain cancers.

What to do:
Melatonin is a natural hormone, but can also be bought and taken as a supplement if levels get too low.

20. Mitochondria

What:
Mitochondria are the powerhouses of the human cell; they convert the energy stored in sugars and fats into adenosine triphosphate (ATP), the essential energy molecule of all animals. ATP is the basic source of energy. It is important for a variety of functions, such as active transport, muscle contraction, and protein synthesis. Although ATP is used for transferring energy, it is not good at storing large amounts of energy for extended periods of time.

Why you care:
Mitochondria are the "engines," or power-generating organelles, of the individual cells of the human body. Not taking care of the mitochondria will

cause a result like an "engine meltdown." They make us "alive" and capable of doing the things we do. They power us up; without them, we could neither live nor function.

What to do:

To protect the mitochondria, it is important to maintain a healthy diet. Being picky about what you eat, and eating less at every meal, will benefit your mitochondria in the long run. Taking supplements such as CoQ10 and Acetyl L-Carnitine can also be of benefit.

22. Protein   *

What:

Protein is a long train of amino acids linked together. Proteins have different functions; they can provide structure (ligaments, fingernails, hair), help in digestion (stomach enzymes), aid in movement (muscles), and play a part in our ability to see (the lens of our eyes is pure crytalline protein). They serve as enzymes, structural elements, hormones, immunoglobulins, etc., and are involved in oxygen transport, muscle contraction, electron transport, and other activities throughout the body.

Why you care:

Our body's structures, functions, and regulation of cells, tissues, and organs cannot exist without proteins. Our muscles, skin, bones, and many other parts of the body contain significant amounts of protein. Protein accounts for 20 percent of total body weight. It is necessary for the building and repair of body tissues and produces enzymes, hormones, and other substances the body uses. It regulates body processes, such as water balancing, transporting nutrients, and making muscles contract. Protein keeps the body healthy by resisting diseases that are common to malnourished people.

What to do:

Protein is available in almost every food. It can also be taken as a supplement or in a health shake. It is recommended to eat approximately 1 gm of protein for every kilogram you weigh per day which is about 0.56 grams per pound.

23. Stem Cells

What:

Adult or somatic stem cells exist throughout the body after embryonic development and are found inside different types of tissue. These stem cells have been found in tissues such as the brain, bone marrow, blood, blood vessels, skeletal muscles, skin, and the liver. They remain in a quiescent or non-dividing state for years until activated by disease or tissue injury.

Why you care:

Adult stem cells can divide or self-renew indefinitely, enabling them to generate a range of cell types from the originating organ or even regenerate the entire original organ. It is generally thought that adult stem cells are limited in their ability to differentiate based on their tissue of origin, but there is some evidence to suggest that they can differentiate to become other cell types.

What to do:

Cord blood banking is the collection and storage of the stem cells found in your newborn's umbilical cord. Today, cord blood stem cells have been used successfully in the treatment of nearly 80 diseases. When you bank your baby's cord blood, you are making a choice that could potentially provide a lifesaving treatment for your child or a family member.

24. Testosterone

What:

Testosterone is a hormone produced by the body. In the early years of a man's life, it is responsible for the normal growth and development of the sex organs, as well as other male physical features such as body hair and muscle development. Normal levels of testosterone contribute to energy, sexual function, mood, and libido. This hormone is necessary for normal male sexual development and functioning; it is also important in maintaining muscle strength and mass.

Why you care:

If your testosterone levels are low, you may have these symptoms: inability to achieve or maintain an erection, decreased sexual desire, fatigue, and depressed mood.

What to do:

To keep your testosterone level up, you will need: vitamins and minerals such as Zinc and vitamin A, B, C, and E, a healthy diet, daily exercise, sexual activity, and adequate sleep.

25. Thyroid

What:

A gland that makes and stores hormones that help regulate the heart rate, blood pressure, body temperature, and the rate at which food is converted into energy. Thyroid hormones are essential for the function of every cell in the body.

Why you care:

They help regulate growth and the rate of chemical reactions (metabolism) in the body. Thyroid hormones also help children grow and develop. The role of the thyroid is to stimulate metabolism and, along with the parathyroid glands (beside or near thyroid), control the body's circulating calcium levels.

What to do:

Iodide is not enough to keep your thyroid healthy. Proper intake of selenium, iron, and essential fatty acids holds the key to a healthy thyroid and metabolism. If you think your thyroid may not be functioning properly, ask your doctor to check your levels.

EXTRAS
26. Triglycerides

What:

Triglycerides are the form in which most fat is stored in the body. Body fat is almost entirely made up of triglycerides. When fat is needed for energy your body releases triglycerides in the form of fatty acids. Triglycerides can come from fat we eat or from excess carbohydrates that are converted to fat.

Why you care:

High triglycerides are an independent risk factor for both heart disease and stroke. An even more important number than your cholesterol level is the ratio of triglycerides to HDL cholesterol. According to research published in Circulation, the Journal of the American Heart Association, and in the journal Clinics, this ratio is a powerful predictor of heart disease.

What to do:

On a low-carb eating plan, triglycerides drop like a rock. This has been seen on virtually every low-carb diet study ever done. The more sugar and carbs you eat, the higher your triglycerides go. High-carb diets raise triglycerides and low-carb diets lower them. It's that simple. Don't eat products that list sugar, fructose, corn syrup, sucrose, dextrose or honey as one of the first ingredients—and try eating more nuts. According to a study in the Archives of Internal Medicine, people with elevated triglycerides were able to lower them by 10 percent by consuming approximately 2 to 3 ounces of nuts a day. Fish oil has also been shown to lower triglycerides, another reason to take this important daily supplement.

27. Vitamin

What:

Vitamins are a group of substances that are essential, in small quantities, for the normal functioning of metabolism in the body. They cannot usually be synthesized in the body, but they occur naturally in certain foods.

Why you care:

Insufficient supply of any particular vitamin results in a deficiency disease. The health benefits of vitamins include their potential ability to prevent various diseases including heart problems, high cholesterol levels, eye disorders, and skin disorders. Most of the vitamins also facilitate the body's mechanisms and perform functions that are not performed by any other nutrient. Vitamins help you regulate body functions and help your body use other nutrients.

What to do:

Maintain a balanced diet consisting of foods with lots of nutrition and use multi-vitamin supplementation.

25 Actions to Speed Up Your Metabolism

Food

1. Graze Like a Sheep

You have probably heard that six small meals a day are better than three larger ones. If you eat frequently, you maintain a higher metabolic rate because the physical act of digestion raises your metabolism. If you only eat one or two times a day, your body goes into starvation mode and stores the food as fat.

2. Eat Your Greens

Three cups of greens a day boosts antioxidants and calcium. You get loads of nutrients for only a few calories.

3. Reduce Your Refined Pastas

Refined pastas are metabolism blockers and send your blood sugar and insulin on a cycle of spiking and crashing all day long. For metabolic success, think about adding protein, such as chicken, to your whole grain pastas.

4. Eat Breakfast

Believe it or not, it may be the most important meal of the day as far as metabolism (and weight loss) is concerned. Breakfast-eaters lose more weight than breakfast-skippers do, according to studies. "Your metabolism slows while you sleep, and it doesn't rev back up until you eat again. So if you bypass breakfast, your body won't burn as many calories until lunchtime as it could. That is why it's smart to start the day with a solid 300-to-400-calorie meal; it jump-starts your metabolism. Aim for a breakfast that has plenty of high-fiber carbs: High-fiber carbohydrates take longer for your body to digest and absorb than simple carbohydrates; thus, they don't cause rapid changes in your blood sugar, so your hunger is kept at bay longer." Some good choices: oatmeal with nuts and berries; whole-grain toast topped with low-fat ricotta and sliced banana or berries; an egg-white veggie omelet with whole-grain toast.

5. Pile on the Protein

Research shows that getting plenty of protein can boost your metabolism, causing you to burn an extra 150 to 200 calories a day. Protein is made up mainly of amino acids, which are harder for your body to break down (than fat and carbs), so you burn more calories getting rid of them. Aim to have a serving of protein at every meal and snack, such as nuts, a small can of tuna, or a piece of low-fat string cheese.

6. Go for "Good" Carbs

Refined carbs, such as bagels, white bread, and potatoes, create a surge in insulin that in turn promotes storage of fat and may drive down your metabolic rate. It is important to keep carbohydrates in your overall diet, but focus on vegetables, fruits, and whole grains, which have less of an impact on insulin levels.

7. Snack Right

Snacking can help ignite your energy by giving your body a fuel boost. Eating healthy snacks, in snack-size portions, can help you avoid the over-hungry/overeating syndrome that often leads to being overweight and can leave you feeling lethargic.

8. Consume Lots of Broccoli!

Study after study links calcium and weight loss. Broccoli is not only high in calcium but also loaded with vitamin C, which boosts calcium absorption.

9. Lean Turkey!

Rev up your fat-burning engine with this bodybuilder favorite. Countless studies have shown that protein can help boost metabolism, lose fat, and build lean muscle tissue so you burn more calories. A 3-ounce serving of boneless, skinless lean turkey breast weighs in at 120 calories and provides 26 grams of appetite-curbing protein, 1 gram of fat, and 0 grams of saturated fat.

10. Reduce Oily Fat Consumption

Increasing metabolism and losing fat is a simple equation. The fact is that you must always burn greater fat than you take in, so start by reducing fatty and oily food (such as certain dressings).

11. Eat Oatmeal!

This heart-healthy favorite ranks high on the good carb list because it is a good source of cholesterol-fighting fiber (7 grams per three-quarter-cup serving) that keeps you full and provides you with the energy you need to make the most of your workouts.

12. Prepare a Light Dinner

Dinner should be your lightest meal. Some experts recommend you not eating anything after 8 p.m. or any later than three to four hours before bedtime. This helps your body process and burn the food when you are awake and moving around and burning more calories per hour.

13. Pick Your Peppers

Take your pick: Jalapenos, chili, cayenne, habanero, etc.—these fiery little guys contain capsaicin, which is why you get a burning sensation in your mouth when you eat them. This same effect is created internally, causing a calorie burn for about 30 minutes afterward. Capsaicin also works as an anti-inflammatory, promoting overall health.

14. Keep Calcium Levels Up

Current obesity research shows that a dip in calcium levels can trigger the same hormone that causes the body to hold on to fat. Choose low-fat dairy, cheese, yogurt, salmon, tofu, and oatmeal.

BEVERAGES

15. Choose Wine for Your Alcohol

Thinking about having a cocktail—or two—before dinner? Think again. Having a drink before a meal causes people to eat around 200 calories more. Drinking with dinner isn't such a good idea either: research has found that the body burns off alcohol first, meaning that the calories in the rest of the meal are more likely to be stored as fat. If you do have a cocktail craving, stick to wine, which packs only 120 calories a glass—or minimize the calories by drinking a white-wine spritzer (two ounces of wine mixed with two ounces of seltzer).

16. DRINK WATER!

Drink half your body weight in ounces every day. For example, if you weigh 160 lbs, aim for 80 oz of water per day. Water is a natural detoxifier in a cup! It will help you get rid of sodium, toxins, and fat. It satisfies cravings, helps you avoid overeating, and gives your system an overall boost.

17. Drink Green Tea

Studies show that green tea extracts boost metabolism and may aid in weight loss. This mood-enhancing tea has also been reported to contain anti-cancer properties and help prevent heart disease.

REST

18. Get Some Shut-eye

Skimping on sleep can derail your metabolism. When you are exhausted, your body lacks the energy to do its normal day-to-day functions, which include burning calories, so your metabolism is automatically lowered. Lack of sleep also increases cortisol levels which can increase belly fat storage.

19. Chill Out!

Long-term stress can make you fat, studies have found. "When you're chronically stressed, your body is flooded with stress hormones, which stimulate fat cells deep in the abdomen to increase in size and encourage fat storage (called toxic weight, because fat deep within your belly is more likely to increase your risk for heart disease, diabetes, and cancer). And stress hormones spark your appetite, making you likely to overeat.

Exercise

20. Do Some Cardio

Cardiovascular exercises, such as walking, jogging, and cycling, are all effective ways to burn calories and keep your metabolism stoked. Exercise 30 to 45 minutes every day. If you are just starting out, use a low-impact, low-intensity exercise such as brisk walking or moderate cycling.

With more experience, you can graduate to jogging or intense group cycling class. Try two-a-day cardio sessions. Breaking up a long workout into two shorter, spaced-out ones burns more calories because of "post-exercise metabolic effect," or the increase in calorie burn for hours after exercise.

21. Increase Daily Activities

Increasing your daily activities not only gives you a higher-level metabolism rate, but also tends to burn more calories. (Good examples: take the stairs, and park far away and walk a bit farther when weather permits.)

22. Pump Some Iron

As we get older, we tend to lose muscle and gain fat—and our metabolism slows down as a result. One way to combat this metabolic slowdown is with regular strength or resistance training. Resistance training stimulates muscles to become stronger and healthier, providing your body with beneficial improvements in strength and function. Resistance training also reduces fat mass and increases muscle mass. Research suggests that resistance training may even increase life expectancy.

23. Incorporate Circuit Training

Without question, you get the most benefit from a combination of strength training and aerobic workouts. Try circuit training to get the benefits of both in half the time! Choose an aerobic exercise (like an elliptical machine). Do 12 minutes of the aerobic exercise, then stop and pick up your resistance bands. Do five minutes of vigorous upper or lower body exercises with the resistance bands. Switch back to your aerobic work for another 12 minutes, and then end with five different resistance band exercises. In 34 minutes, you incorporated both types of exercises, burning calories and fat, and building lean muscle!

24. Stand, Walk, and Move

Keep your metabolism revved up with small, frequent movements like tapping your feet, rolling your neck in circles, or shrugging your shoulders. If you sit for long periods of time, try to get up at least once an hour to walk around and stretch.

25. Try Yoga

By building muscle through body weight resistance, yoga helps to strengthen and tone muscles. It has also been shown to boost metabolism by stimulating the thyroid gland and lowering cortisol levels.

25 Tools for Your Ultimate Health Tool Chest

#	Tool	Why	Price
1.	Blood pressure arm band	Monitor your blood pressure levels	$60
2.	Body ball / exercise ball	Balance / flexibility exercise tool	$20
3.	Calipers	Track your progress	$50
4.	CrossCore War Machine	Resistance exercise tool	$250
5.	Dumbbell set	Resistance exercise tool	$300
6.	FitBit	Track your steps, activity, and sleep	$99
7.	Foam roller	Roll out sore muscles	$25
8.	Food scale	Monitor portion size	$25
9.	Glass / stainless steel water bottle	Keeps you hydrated and safe from toxins found in plastic and synthetic bottles	$15
10.	Heart strap / watch	Monitor your calorie burn	$70
11.	Jump rope	Cardio exercise tool	$10
12.	Kettle bell	Resistance exercise tool	$40
13.	Medicine ball	Resistance exercise tool	$20
14.	Mini trampoline	Cardio exercise tool	$50
15.	Pull-up bar	Resistance exercise tool	$30
16.	Punching bag / boxing gloves	Cardio exercise tool	$150
17.	Road bicycle	Cardio exercise tool	$200
18.	Speed ladder	Cardio exercise tool	$25
19.	Stationary bike	Cardio exercise tool	$200
20.	Step equipment	Cardio exercise tool	$35
21.	Tape measure	Keep track of your progress	$10
22.	Treadmill	Cardio exercise tool	$250
23.	Weight scale	Monitor your weight	$45
24.	Xertube resistance band	Resistance exercise tool	$10
25.	Yoga mat	Flexibility exercise tool	$20

Section III - Health Tools

Health Tools

Ultimate Health Matrix

What It Is	Why It Matters	How to Maximize Actions
HORMONES		
Cortisol	Adrenal hormone produced in response to stress or anxiety In excess, can increase blood pressure and blood sugar levels In excess, can decrease immune response and increase weight gain	Consume lean proteins and healthy (Omega-3) fats Minimize high-gluten and high-GI foods Exercise regularly Decrease stress
DHEA	Precursor to sex hormones, produced by the adrenals Converted into androgens in males Converted into estrogens in females	Restrict caloric intake Exercise regularly Reduce mental/emotional stress
Dopamine	Affects mood and pleasure sensitivity Helps regulate emotional responses and decision-making Low levels can lead to depression, cravings, addictions, low sex drive, and inability to focus	Eat foods rich in complex carbohydrates Make sure you are getting enough tryptophan and B6 in your diet
Estrogen	Primary female sex hormone Promotes growth and development Affects metabolism and tissue function Linked to mood disruptions May support prostate health in men	Increase consumption of cruciferous vegetables (broccoli, cauliflower, cabbage, greens, etc.) Get enough folic acid Exercise regularly
Gastrin	Aids in digestion	Undergo testing if you have symptoms of an ulcer
Ghrelin and Leptin	Stimulates hunger and indicates satiation	Consume lean proteins, healthy fats, and low-GI complex carbohydrates Minimize high-sugar foods
Growth Hormone	Made by the pituitary gland; essential for healthy growth Affects metabolism and energy May help slow the aging process	Consult your physician to determine whether a supplement is needed
HCG	Hormone produced during pregnancy An elevated level (when not pregnant) can indicate the presence of cancer May work to suppress hunger and promote fat-burning	Consult your physician to determine if hormone testing is necessary

What It Is	Why It Matters	How to Maximize Actions
Insulin	Regulates carbohydrate and fat metabolism Causes cells to utilize glucose in the blood When control of insulin levels fails, diabetes occurs	Substitute simple carbohydrates (high-sugar foods) for low GI, complex carbohydrates Minimize consumption of fruit juices and sodas
Melatonin	Helps control your sleep and wake cycle Promotes healthy, natural sleep	Consult your physician to determine whether a supplement is needed
Progesterone	Important sex hormone for females Helps balance against too much estrogen Primary hormone of fertility and pregnancy	Consume foods high in B6 Minimize processed foods Try to eat only hormone-free meats
Serotonin	Regulates intestinal movements Promotes healthy mood, appetite, and sleep cycles Low levels often result in depression	Get plenty of exercise— and rest Eat a balanced diet that minimizes high-GI foods
Testosterone	Important sex hormone Promotes development of muscle mass Helps strengthen bones Contributes to energy level and overall health	Consume high-quality proteins Increase consumption of healthy fats Minimize "bad" fats Limit alcohol intake Add zinc, magnesium, B6, and Vitamin C to your diet
Thyroid (T3 and T4)	Regulate cell functions for entire body Act as messengers for cells Facilitates metabolism	Consume healthy whole foods rich in iodine and antioxidants Minimize glutenous and high-sugar foods Get plenty of exercise
VITAMINS		
A	Promotes healthy vision Helps promote healthy immune system	Incorporate organ meats, eggs, and dairy products into your diet Eat plenty of dark, colorful vegetables (carrots, sweet potatoes, etc.)
B1 (Thiamine)	Helps maintain energy supplies Coordinates activity of muscles and nerves Supports healthy heart function	Consume plenty of vegetables such as asparagus, crimini mushrooms, spinach, green peas, and brussels sprouts
B2 (Riboflavin)	Helps the body convert food into fuel (glucose) to produce energy Helps the body use oxygen and create red blood cells	Find B2 in liver, dairy products, and green leafy vegetables
B3 (Niacin)	Helps the body make various sex and stress-related hormones Helps improve circulation Helps lower LDL and triglyceride levels	Find B3 in beets, beef liver, fish, sunflower seeds, and peanuts

What It Is	Why It Matters	How to Maximize Actions
B5 (Pantothenic acid)	Helps provide energy Promotes healthy adrenal gland functioning May help slow the aging process	Find B5 in beef, eggs, legumes, mushrooms, and nuts
B6 (Pyridoxine)	Necessary for breakdown and synthesis of amino acids Aids in metabolism Maintains central nervous system Helps lower stress and depression	Find B6 in lean meats, fish, most vegetables, nuts, and whole grains
B9 (Folic Acid)	Synthesizes DNA and RNA Aids cell division, growth, and repair Produces red blood cells Enhances brain health	Consume plenty of whole grains and green leafy vegetables
B12	Promotes healthy red blood cell formation, neurological function, and DNA synthesis	Be sure to eat plenty of fish, shellfish, eggs, lean meat, and dairy products
C (Ascorbic acid)	Essential for normal growth and repair of the body's cells and tissues Helps prevent damage to cells caused by free radicals	Consume plenty of fresh fruits and vegetables (especially citrus fruits)
D	Promotes bone health Helps prevent serious diseases such as cancer, diabetes, and heart disease Aids in the absorption of calcium	Be sure to get enough exposure to sunlight (with proper precautions like sunscreen) Check your level. Find Vitamin D in fish, eggs, fortified milk, and cod liver oil
E	Protects body tissue from damage of oxidation Plays an important role in cell-signaling mechanisms Helps prevent premature aging	Incorporate avocados, nuts, asparagus, olive oil, and leafy vegetables into your diet
K	Promotes healthy blood clotting Helps build strong bones Helps prevent heart disease and cancer	Find Vitamin K in green leafy vegetables and fermented foods (like natto and tempeh)
MINERALS		
Boron	Helps minimize bone loss and alleviate arthritis Aids in synthesis of calcium	Consume plenty of fruit, vegetables, and nuts
Calcium	Crucial for healthy bones, muscles, and nerve conduction	Consume plenty of dairy products and vegetables Consult your physician to determine whether a supplement is needed
Chromium	Helps regulate blood sugar and insulin levels	Find it in liver, whole grain cereals, lean meat, eggs, and cheese

What It Is	Why It Matters	How to Maximize Actions
Copper	Promotes healthy function of nervous and cardiovascular systems Promotes healthy immune and reproductive systems Helps protect against harmful germs and bacteria	Incorporate sesame seeds, cashews, and sunflower seeds into your diet
Iodine	Essential for normal growth and development Helps regulate the rate of energy production	Find it in cod, yogurt, iodized salt
Iron	Transports oxygen throughout body Promotes healthy immune system Helps body produce energy	Find it in beef, fish, poultry, spinach, asparagus, romaine lettuce, tofu, greens, and broccoli Supplement if tendancy toward anemia
Manganese	Promotes strong and healthy bones Helps maintain normal blood sugar levels Aids in protein metabolism	Find it in mustard greens, raspberries, spinach, pineapple, brown rice, garlic, grapes, and tofu
Magnesium	Helps maintain normal muscle and nerve function Supports healthy immune system Promotes strong and healthy bones	Find it in green leafy vegetables, nuts, and whole grains
Molybdenum	Controls movement and release of iron in the body Helps transport oxygen Aids enzyme function	Find it in beans, beef liver, cereal grains, green leafy vegetables, and legumes
Nickel	Activates liver enzymes Promotes strong and healthy bones	Find it in dark chocolate, nuts, beans, peas, shellfish, and grains
Phosphorus	Builds healthy bones and teeth Improves digestion and excretion	Find it in milk, dairy products, meat, fish, whole grains, and green leafy vegetables
Potassium	Promotes proper heart function Helps regulate fluid levels Aids in protein synthesis	Incorporate sweet potatoes, bananas, prunes, and spinach into your diet
Selenium	Promotes healthy thyroid function Helps maintain healthy muscles Contributes to proper energy levels	Incorporate Brazil nuts, crab, fish, and liver into your diet
Silicon	Strengthens bones and connective tissues Promotes healthy hair, skin, and nails	Find it in apples, unrefined grains, almonds, and honey
Sodium	Facilitates enzyme operation and muscle contraction Contributes to blood regulation Helps regulate fluid levels	Since it is found in many foods (especially when prepared), guard against over-consumption

What It Is	Why It Matters	How to Maximize Actions
Tin	Helps protein synthesis May help decrease depression and fatigue	Find it in canned goods Proper levels can be maintained through a basic balanced diet
Vanadium	Strengthens bones and teeth	Find it in radishes, mushrooms, parsley, and grains
Zinc	Promotes proper functioning of immune system, metabolism, digestion, and energy levels	Find it in oysters, turnips, pumpkin seeds, oats, and meat
CRITICAL SUCCESS FACTORS		
Blood pressure	A high blood pressure exposes you to significant health risks including: heart disease, heart attack, congestive heart failure, and stroke	Maintain a healthy, balanced diet Get plenty of regular exercise and rest Reduce stress
Cholesterol	High cholesterol is a major risk factor for heart disease, heart attack, and stroke	Get plenty of regular exercise and rest Consume a diet low in saturated fats Work with your physician to maintain proper levels
Glucose	High/unstable blood sugar levels lead to overeating, and long-term, to diabetes	Minimize high-GI foods Exercise regularly
Protein	Proteins are the building blocks of body tissues	Consume plenty of healthy, lean meats, dairy products, nuts, and legumes
Triglycerides	High levels contribute to the hardening of arteries and thickening of artery walls Increases risk of heart disease, heart attack, and stroke	Exercise regularly Eliminate trans fats Minimize high-GI foods Limit alcohol consumption
Uric acid	High levels can lead to gout or kidney diseases	Limit caffeine and alcohol consumption Drink plenty of water

Ultimate Health VIPs

CHAPTER 1 – LIFESTYLE

Assessment:

How are you living your life? Managing balance, managing risks, resting, saying "no" enough, and getting enough exercise all make up your overall living routine. Are your habits supporting your health?

VIPs:

1. Your lifestyle determines your longevity.
2. Exercise is medicine.
3. There are three types of aging: chronological, mental, and physical. Ultimate Health includes managing the way you age.
4. Research suggests that you can alter the effects of aging with diet, chemical management, exercise, and preventive activities.
5. Making time in your busy schedule for exercise and stress relief/relaxation is paramount.

CHAPTER 2 – MENTAL MANAGEMENT

Assessment:

What goes on in our minds truly impacts our health. Assess your self-talk, your daily attitude, your beliefs about being healthy and not getting sick, and your willingness to release grudges and forgive, while focusing on the positives. Filter the input you receive from sources such as news, media, or even negative people.

VIPs:

1. Mental management is a crucial aspect of Ultimate Health.
2. You are what you think! Think positive, healthy thoughts and affirmations.
3. Be intentional; surround yourself with positive people, images, places, and things to increase your mental health, outcomes, and results.
4. Continually learn and grow to develop your mind and soul. Consistently add new experiences and inspiration to your world.

5. Make every room you enter a happier place in part because you are there.

CHAPTER 3 – ULTIMATE LONGEVITY

Assessment:

Do you have a great team of health professionals that know you and guide you? Family doctor? Nutritionist? Dentist? Do you have regular checkups and vaccines? Do your behaviors align with real health?

VIPs:

1. Having a strong team that acts as a positive support system to help you stay ahead of the curve is a major step toward disease management.
2. The difference between healthcare and sick care is proactive testing, prevention, and a holistic mind-set. Be smart and proactive; work to maintain your health.
3. Look and feel ten years younger with disease prevention, screening, and developing an Ultimate Health plan with your health team.
4. Get your preventive blood work analyzed at least once a year and make adjustments where needed.

CHAPTER 4 – ELIMINATING STRESS

Assessment:

Are you managing anxiety? Are you meditating? Relaxing enough? Is your life aligned with your values? Have you set up harmony in your life so things run as smoothly as possible? Is your pace of life contributing to or detracting from your overall well-being?

VIPs:

1. Your true wealth is determined by the amount of things you do not have to worry about.
1. Identify your stressors . . . then begin eliminating them!
3. Detox your life from negative people, places, and things.
4. Create systems for organization, values clarification, and completion.
5. Build margin time into your days, schedules, and calendaring.

6. When issues arise, ask yourself often, "does it really matter?" Calm down, breathe, and relax.

CHAPTER 5 – STRENGTHENING YOUR IMMUNE SYSTEM

Assessment:

Your immune system protects you. It detects potential harm and helps your body react. Are you helping yourself? Are you resting at the right time—for example, when you sense your body needs it to ensure you stay well? Are you maintaining good hygiene, protecting against harmful bacteria, practicing plain and simple cleanliness such as washing your hands enough, and avoiding being in contact with the wrong things in order to support your wellness?

VIPs:

1. Reduce stress to strengthen your immune system.
2. Research, become aware of, and choose immune system-boosting foods!
3. Vaccines against microorganisms that cause diseases can prepare the body's immune system and help fight—or prevent—an infection.
4. Utilize meditation, music, prayer, and anything else that positively contributes to your spiritual and emotional well-being in order to help boost your body's natural immune system (including proper rest).
5. Wash your hands often and keep your environment as clean as possible.
6. Maintaining cardiovascular fitness through regular exercise has been shown to be a significant immune booster.

CHAPTER 6 – PREVENTIVE TESTING

Assessment:

Early detection is great common sense in today's world of information. How is your discipline on staying current on screenings, blood work reviews, EKGs, MRIs, hormones testing, and urinalysis—even full-body skin screenings every few years? There are many simple things we can do to be proactive. Are you taking advantage of these options?

VIPs:

1. Preventive testing saves—and extends—lives.
2. You can live as though you were physically many years younger simply through early detection, planning, and troubleshooting in order to prevent disease.
3. Know your numbers! Get your cholesterol, hormones, and blood tested annually and as often as optimal for Ultimate Health maintenance.
4. Sharing your family history with your health team can help to assess risk factors and formulate a proactive plan.

CHAPTER 7 – EXERCISE, MOVEMENT, AND LONGEVITY

Assessment:

Physical exercise matters—regular, frequent, and ongoing. Strength resistance, cardiovascular exercise (aerobics), balance, and stretching all promote a better-operating body.

VIPs:

1. Many overlook the fact that all four types of exercise should be in most people's routine: resistance, cardio, stretching, and balance.
2. Effective exercise is one of the single most important things you can do for your body.
3. When you engage in physical activity such as running, biking, yoga, or weight training, you increase your heart rate and can really super-turbo-charge your metabolism!
4. High-intensity interval training (like running short sprints) also boosts metabolism and requires minimal time commitment.
5. Resistance training activates muscles all over your body and increases your average daily metabolic rate. Yet another reason to pump iron!

CHAPTER 8 – ORAL HEALTH

Assessment:

Obviously, it is important to keep your mouth clean. Are you brushing enough? Flossing enough? Going for regular checkups?

VIPs:

1. Oral health can significantly impact your overall health.
2. Emerging research has shed a harsh light on the dangerous link between gum disease and heart health.
3. To protect your oral health, resolve to practice good oral hygiene every day.
4. Watch for signs and symptoms of oral disease and contact your dentist as soon as a problem arises.
5. Get regular cleanings and annual checkups.

CHAPTER 9 – VISION CARE

Assessment:

Are you protecting your eyes from sunlight and eating the things that help prevent cataracts later in life? Are you going for regular checkups? Do you wear eye protection when doing certain types of work around the house? All these factors add up to promoting this key component to your body's overall health.

VIPs:

1. Anything good for heart, skin, and blood vessel health is also good for your eyes.
2. Like other parts of the body, the cornea and retina of the eye are protected by the antioxidants in fresh fruits and vegetables; eat plenty!
3. Exercise has been shown to promote brain health, function, and renewal. Since the eye is part of the brain, this exercise benefit has been found to extend to ocular tissues as well.
4. Eye exams should be performed on an annual basis.
5. Be safe and protect your eyes with sunglasses and protection gear when working or being around dangerous activities.

CHAPTER 10 – TOXIN ELIMINATION

Assessment:

What's around you can get in your body through your skin, what you breathe, and what you eat. Toxins are potentially hazardous substances that can place an extra toll on your body such as forcing your liver and kidneys to work overtime as they filter fluids. Are you protecting yourself like you could or should?

VIPs:

1. Remember: chemical toxins exist in the food we eat, the grass we walk on, and the air we breathe.
2. Toxins can also include any negative or harmful event, thought, emotion, substance, or habit that has the potential to affect your performance or life.
3. Do your best to live in Ultimate Health by eliminating toxins and opting for organic foods, surrounding yourself with great people, and maintaining clean environments.

CHAPTER 11 – HORMONES

Assessment:

A hormone is a chemical released by a cell or a gland in one part of your body that sends out messages that affect cells in other parts of your body. In essence, it's a chemical messenger that transports a signal from one cell to another. Have you tested your chemical balances (estrogen, testosterone, thyroid, DHEA, etc.)? Are you supplementing where you should or could or do you have some blind spots?*

VIPs:

1. Our hormones work in concert with physical fitness, good nutrition, proper sleep, and stress reduction/spiritual wellness to produce a symphony of Ultimate Health.
2. Hormones are messengers of the body.
3. Most people begin losing optimal production of many hormones at or around age 30 and fail to take action to adjust, thereby preventing their

body from operating at peak performance.

4. Testosterone is an example of an important hormone. Low testosterone could be behind a lethargic sex drive, brain fog, and lower metabolism.

5. Doing annual blood labs and studying your hormone levels with your health team to ensure optimal ranges can have magnificent results on your body's functioning and aging.

6. Taking care of your hormones is important for everyone—not just for women during menopause.

7. Low thyroid levels are frequently the cause of persistent fatigue, constant coldness, and female hair loss, and may contribute to depression.

CHAPTER 12 – VITAMINS

Assessment:

A vitamin is an organic compound required as a vital nutrient in tiny amounts by an organism. Vitamins help your body function optimally. Are you managing your regular intake, testing so you know, and living daily with the right balances in your body?

VIPs:

1. Many vitamins are deficient in people's bodies. At a minimum, a strong, daily multiple vitamin is just good, simple practice.

2. Vitamin C is a powerful antioxidant that helps to fight against cancer and heart disease. Citrus fruits, berries, dark leafy greens, and peppers are natural sources.

3. Vitamin D has huge benefits and can be obtained through sunlight and other sources. Some studies have shown that up to 80 percent of Americans have substantial to very unhealthy low levels of Vitamin D.

4. CoQ10 assists in maintaining good cardiovascular health and may slow the progression of Alzheimer's. Organ meats, fish, sesame, and grape seed oils are all excellent sources.

CHAPTER 13 – CALORIC MANAGEMENT

Assessment:

A calorie is a unit of energy. It is a measure of the energy we generate with every task we do, as well as a measure of the energy delivered by a food we eat. How well do you know your body and how you balance what you eat versus what you need to perform? Being in tune and knowing this can allow you to make better daily choices . . . and live better!

VIPs:

1. By understanding how your body processes foods and burns calories, you can become slimmer, trimmer, and fitter this year than you were a decade ago.

2. Educating yourself about the foods and energy you provide your body is a very important step toward Ultimate Health. Not all calories are created equal!

3. Overall, caloric restriction is one of the best ways to lose weight and keep it off if you can maintain a lower caloric restriction. The average person uses between 1,500 and 2,000 calories on an average day. A pound of fat stores about 3,500 calories, and in order to lose a pound of fat, you need to burn an extra 3,500 calories. To lose a pound in one week, that would mean creating a calorie deficit of 500 calories per day with diet, exercise, or both. That is why when we reduce calories and stay sedentary, not much happens. Not all calories are created equal. Some help your body strive while others leave you craving more. Take care in the foods you choose.

4. One key to controlling your metabolism and hunger is educating yourself about the glycemic index (GI) of the carbohydrates in your diet. Foods with a high GI are rapidly digested and result in large increases in blood sugar. They also tend to cause a rapid decline in blood sugar, which leads to fatigue after eating them. Foods with a low GI are digested more slowly and cause a more gradual rise in blood sugar and insulin release. These have proven to decrease weight gain and improve performance. Maintaining low levels of insulin is important to allow your body to tap into stored fat for fuel.

5. Knowledge can enhance your life. Read labels to increase your awareness of excess sugar and salt in many processed foods.

CHAPTER 14 – EARS, NOSE, AND THROAT

Assessment:

Preventive testing is important for the ear, nose, and throat, the same as for the rest of your body. It is important to protect your hearing and ear canal from foreign objects and loud noises. Are you maintaining good hygiene? Are you getting checked regularly?

VIPs:

1. Preventive testing is important for the ear, nose, and throat, as well as for the rest of your body.
2. Foreign substance in the ear or nose should be treated by the proper medical expert.
3. It is important to protect your hearing and ear canal from foreign objects and loud noises.

CHAPTER 15 – NUTRITION

Assessment:

Food is any substance consumed to provide nutritional support for your body. It is usually of plant or animal origin, and contains essential nutrients, such as carbohydrates, fats, proteins, vitamins, and minerals. It is what we consume in an effort to produce energy, maintain life, and stimulate growth. How is your balance? Are you eating throughout the day to promote good metabolism? Do you eat slowly and really chew well in order to promote good digestion? Do you make healthy choices such as limiting the fried, processed, and high-sugar foods you eat?

VIPs:

1. Food is medicine. Eat healthily at meals—and consistently every few hours throughout the day.
2. Fresh, organic berries and colorful vegetables are a great choice whether at home or dining out. They contain potent antioxidants that help prevent cancer by fighting free radicals.
3. Avoid sugars and simple carbohydrates. They are burned quickly and can lead to increased cravings.

CHAPTER 16 – SKIN HEALTH

Assessment:

Your skin is the largest organ in your body. It acts as an external filter and can even provide many clues about the condition of your body internally. Are you protecting it like you should from ultraviolet rays and from harmful chemicals that can get into your body? Do you get body screenings to detect cancers or other harmful things that need attention in order to ensure your Ultimate Health?

VIPs:

1. Sunscreen is needed year-round for protection against harmful rays.
2. Vitamin D can actually come from the sun and may affect moods when deficient. This crucial hormone assists all systems of the body.
3. With proper nutrition, sunscreen, and skin care, you can reduce the effects of aging and increase a youthful glow.
4. Every one to two years, have a dermatologist do a full-body skin screening for early detection of skin-related abnormalities.

CHAPTER 17 – FLUIDS

Assessment:

Consuming adequate amounts of water is critical to maintaining Ultimate Health. Do you drink enough water each day? Do you manage your alcohol intake? Do you drink too much soda or other high-sugar drinks?

VIPs:

1. Keep your body well hydrated.
2. Beware of the hidden calories in fruit juices and sodas.
3. Often, hunger is mistaken for thirst. One glass of water can make you feel full and help stave off hunger cravings!
4. Carefully manage alcohol intake. When under the influence of alcohol, a person often makes bad eating choices (among others) that can impact health and increase risk.

CHAPTER 18 – MANAGING YOUR EMOTIONS

Assessment:

Emotion is a complex psycho-physiological experience of your state of mind as you interact with internal and external influences. How is your mood, temperament, disposition, and motivation? All these elements matter; all impact the way our bodies perform.

VIPs:

1. Managing your emotions is critical to Ultimate Health.
2. Everyone is different. Be intentional about eliminating the things that make you feel negative—and increasing the things that make you feel positive!
3. If you are not seeing the world, your job, or your life in a positive light—make changes!

CHAPTER 19 – SLEEP

Assessment:

Sleep suspends the sensory activity of nearly all voluntary muscles. It accentuates the growth and rejuvenation of the immune, nervous, skeletal, and muscular systems. Are you getting enough sleep? Is it good sleep?

VIPs:

1. Be intentional about getting more sleep.
2. Diets (calorie restricted) for weight loss are much more likely to fail with chronic sleep loss.
3. Limit alcohol, caffeine, and heavy meals late in the day.
4. Utilize natural solutions that encourage sleep: quieting the mind, exercise, melatonin, a warm bath, soothing scents, music.
5. Start viewing sleep as a tool to elevate your lifestyle and give you more energy during the day.

CHAPTER 20 – SPIRITUAL WELLNESS

Assessment:

Your spiritual wellness is to a large degree reflective of your worldview. Is it egocentric or others oriented? Would others say you display stress tolerance and adequate marginal reserves for life's challenges? What wisdom do you apply to your life situations in order to achieve spiritual balance, peace and joy?

VIPs:

1. Spiritual wellness derives from maintaining margin and boundaries, seeking soul enrichment, and reaching out to give to others.

2. The American trend of seeking primarily financial wealth, pleasure, personal peace, and avoidance of pain is not a reflection of spiritual wholeness.

3. Your life is a mix of body, mind, and spirit. If you ignore one aspect, you will feel stress and be out of balance in one or both of the other two.

4. Invest in your spiritual side and nourish your soul by reading and spending time alone in prayer and meditation—every day!

*The most important thing you can do to get results
is to get clarity about your health. I teach these same
principles in my studio with clients. Once you have clarity, focus,
and execution, you're rolling.*
—Tony Jeary

TONY JEARY

Tony Jeary - The RESULTS Guy™, often referred to as the Coach to the World's Top CEOs and High Achievers has been positively impacting lives of the most successful, for over 20 years.

His signature best selling book "Strategic Acceleration, Success at the Speed of Life" has 3 foundation secrets Tony shares daily through his Success columns, *RESULTS* magazine, books and keynotes... Clarity, Focus and Execution. He believes strongly in all three of these simple yet powerful words... and all three have led him to co-author this book, for you.

Tony is a goal setter who makes things happen. He's helped many, many do the same and achieve extraordinary results both personally and professionally. In 2010, he discovered (with Clarity) that many of his high achieving clients truly wanted to have better health and welcomed his help. They wanted to know what to focus on so they could live in "Ultimate Health". So...

Tony went on a crusade. He began studying everything he could on what mattered most regarding health. The real, what he calls HLA s (High Leverage Activities). He decided to live out and prove out everything in this book. He went from 202 lbs, 38 inch waist, 24% body fat with a tad of high blood pressure to 162 lbs, 32 inch waist and 11% body fat, with ideal vitals all around including perfect blood pressure.

With this new knowledge, and with this personal track record, he teamed up his doctor, Rick Wilson who opened Tony's eyes of what's possible along with Dr Engles and his good friend Tammy Kling and built this quick read book.

Today, Tony works from his private Strategic Acceleration Studio on his estate in DFW, Texas where he coaches and strategizes with top performers on how they can think smarter and accelerate their business and personal results including inspiring them to live healthy.

Please visit www.tonyjeary.com or www.strategicacceleration.com for more details on how Tony Jeary International can impact your organization and your life.

Tony Jeary

Before fitness and health transformation

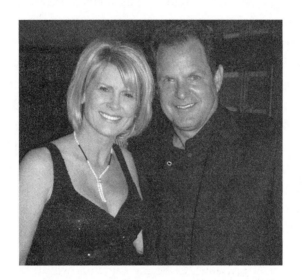

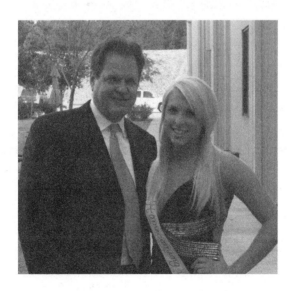

TONY JEARY
After

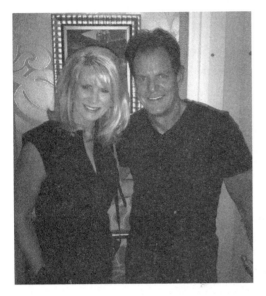

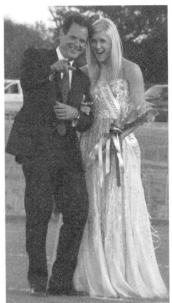

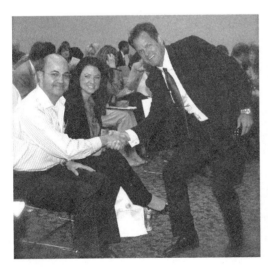

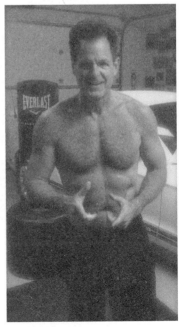

DR. RICK WILSON

Dr. Rick Wilson, MD, has worked with patients in creating healthy lives, habits, and mindsets, for decades.

He currently practices at the Cooper Clinic in Dallas, Texas. Dr. Wilson is a renowned speaker and author interested in saving lives. He enjoys sharing with audiences on a variety of proactive topics including:

- Living in ultimate health
- Your Longevity Power: exercise and preventive medicine testing
- The importance of sun protection and anti-aging skin care habits for longevity and appearance
- Hormones and the vital role they play in your life

Dr. Wilson is available to speak to corporate audiences about overall health and wellness.

RICK WILSON

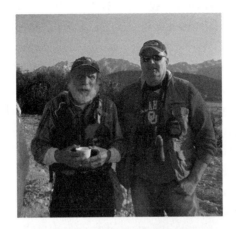

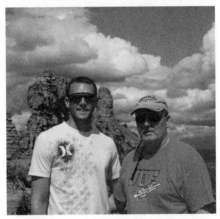

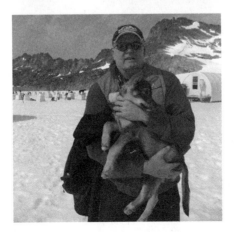

JENNIFER ENGELS, MD

Jennifer Engels, MD is a diagnostic radiologist in the Dallas Fort Worth area who has a special interest in disease prevention, nutrition, and early intervention.

Her motivation for helping others is her life's work with patients.

Reading abnormal body imaging scans for many years was frustrating and became a catalyst to help others. Jennifer desires to help others transform their lives and is determined to try to prevent disease or at least catch it early while it is still curable.

Jennifer has received an additional degree in integrative nutrition and health coaching in order to help educate and empower patients to prevent diseases and reach their ultimate health.

Jennifer Engels

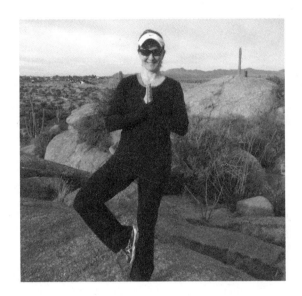

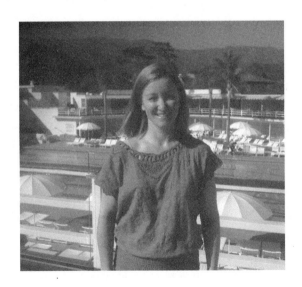

Tammy Kling

Tammy Kling is an international best selling author and publishing coach of 101 books.

She has appeared on Dateline NBC, The Discovery Channel, Primetime 20/20, Oprah, Geraldo, and in The New York Times and Wall Street Journal.

Tammy specializes in ghostwriting corporate books that transform cultures and help build brands, sell companies, or manage messaging through online identity management, and book distribution to global prospects and clients.

As CEO of The Writer's Group, a hybrid company that merges those in need with work projects, Tammy helps corporate CEO's and entrepreneurs fulfill a lifelong dream. The Writers group is an international group of writers that builds websites, PR packages, blogs, story boards and books. They use words, to change lives. Tammy has collaborated on books with corporations, non-profits, speakers, athletes, and entrepreneurs. She is also the founder of the homeless writers project - a filming, literary, and homeless speakers program to help rehabilitate and inspire the homeless.

Tammy's desire to use words to change lives, began in the jungle of Colombia when she was a Crisis Management Team Leader with a major airline, working with families in search of their loved ones after a crash. In the quest for survivors her first book, Exit Row, was born. This book was recently featured in a segment on aviation on the Discovery Channel and Tammy has lectured on crisis management at Universities across the world.

Inside today's corporations, Tammy coaches employees and teams in crisis management and stress reduction as part of corporate wellness initiatives. Tammy has written several books with CEOs of companies on total life prosperity and physical and emotional wellness, including Dr. Wayne Andersen's Optimal Health, and Viverae Corporations book, Working to Live.

Companies she's worked inside include: ESPN, Lululemon, American Airlines, Wrigley, Dial, and the National Forest Service among others. If you'd like Tammy to help make your brand, website or book dreams become a reality contact her at tammykling@me.com

Tammy Kling

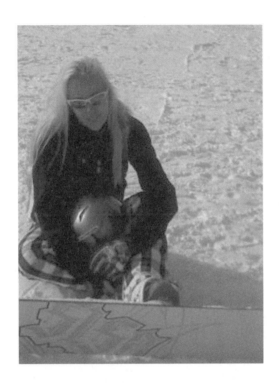

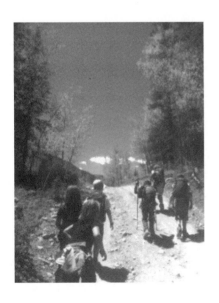

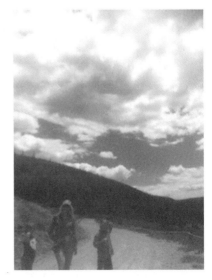

Call to Action

Final words to encourage you
in your own life....

We collaborated on this work to impact lives.

Throughout this process it evolved into more of a research project centered around health, and all the ways you can become better emotionally, physically, and spiritually. We spent months with doctors in various fields. We listened, asked questions, and field tested their advice, supplements, and healthy habit recommendations.

We printed many review copies and sent books to special selected people to have them help us tweak, improve, confirm accuracy and catch anything that might make the book more impactful for you the reader. During this process, several of our pre-readers and clients, communicated back that they felt our readers would really want to know more about how to tangibly apply these Ultimate Health principles to their own lives. Specifically, many just wanted to know - how do you lose weight in the healthiest way? How do you lose ten pounds, and keep it off? There are a ton of diet books on the market. And, every doctor we have been privileged to work with during this process had a lot of different suggestions and theories but the commonality is exercise and diet!

Everyone agrees that food is medicine.

Each one of us has had varied experiences regarding health and fitness. Tony lost 40 pounds, and changed his mindset, which was the catalyst for this book. Tammy lost 50 pounds of baby weight she had gained while she was pregnant with her first child, and lost it through calorie restriction and taking up a new sport - running. Much to her surprise, she gained a passion for running and lost all 50 pounds in six weeks. Today she runs trails and participates in mountain runs with her kids. Her passion for running evolved into the adventure blog - escape suburbia. Doctors Jen and Rick are both active, and desire to encourage others to live healthy and avoid common medical afflictions such as metabolic syndrome. Dr. Wilson actively works in two resistive workouts and three cardio workouts every week, despite his busy schedule, seeing patients. So as we discussed our own views on health, we thought it would be important to show what Tony did personally to transform his, because it was the catalyst for this book. As he changed, he began to help change his clients' mindsets towards health. All that evolved into a different way of living.

IN HIS OWN WORDS:

How I lost 40 pounds, reduced body fat, and altered my thinking to live in Ultimate Health:

1. I got inspired by 2 others in my life who changed, like I'm hoping I inspire you to do.

2. I found a smart doctor who lives and has studied preventative health, and that's Dr Rick my doctor and co-author

3. I then went on a search to find others to help me learn more about nutrition, diet and how the body really works, like Dr Engels and others on my team

4. I learned healthy habits such as:

    A. Careful food choices every single day (out with candy, fufu drinks, fried foods etc. All bad food and drinks gone forever. See our list of 25 foods to avoid and 25 to eat) Manage my calories and front load the day with the most calories starting at breakfast.

    B. Chemistry managment of my body (consistent lab work, and careful, calculated supplements accordingly for ideal levels of hormones, vitamins, minerals)

    C. Exercise daily, simple everyday exercise mostly for me in my home gym area, with weights, rubber bands, stretching, balance, walking and bike rides.

    D. Sleep more... 8 hrs a day AND less stress, saying no more and asking myself "does it really matter?"

    E. A clear vision of my goals... words and pictures everywhere around my life so I can see who I wanted to become and I could measure my progress having my coaches/ trainers and others around me support me, encourage me and help me be accountable.

As you can see, Tony's steps are not earth shattering or unattainable.

However, it does require clarity, focus and execution, the three principles he teaches business leaders!

Diet isn't a four letter word

It has become popular in our culture to think of the word diet, as a bad thing. But weight gain is linked to major disease such as diabetes, stroke, and coronary disease. Excess weight, and obesity, is the cause of death and disability for millions of people! Does diet still sound like a bad word? A diet is simply something you do to lose excess weight. Then, it's important to practice continual daily healthy habits to keep your weight where it should be, and increase fitness.

Want to drop those final ten pounds?

Dr. Rick Wilson offers this specific three point action plan for successful weight loss, as endorsed by a Cooper Clinic Registered Dietitian:

3 points to success:
1. Portion control
2. Regular meals - no skipping early in the day & then gorging later. This has to do with blood sugar control and subsequent cravings. If we have one or two healthy (fruit, etc.) snacks spread between breakfast & lunch and then lunch & dinner, we don't have the big insulin & high-to-low blood sugar swings which drive cravings. So caloric restriction is fine, as long as you're not starving yourself!
3. Beware of hidden calories! Watch out for calorie-laden drinks --- those lattes, soft drinks, etc. add up to lots of wasted calories --- and alcoholic beverages. Consume more (9-13) servings of quality (organic) fresh fruits and vegetables. Just say no to fruit drinks and soda.

Remember, we created this book to help give you an awareness of the simplest steps you can take to develop the habits that will lead to ultimate health. Part of this knowledge is understanding your body, and your blood and how it all works together.

These three steps above generally lower your glycemic load and the big swings of insulin.

***Interesting note: sleep deprivation plays a big role in our appetite choic-

es, as it drives you to seek more rapidly stimulating sugary and fatty foods for quick energy and the abused stimulants (such as 5 Hour Energy) drinks that are unhealthy for you.

As you add these three steps to your day, don't forget to get your beauty sleep! You'll feel more energized, sharper at work, mentally focused, and physically strong.

Ultimate Health Results Corporate Wellness Seminar

Half-day

Dr. Rick Wilson: 7 Keys to Healthy Longevity
Dr. Jennifer Engels: Metabolic awareness for health

Dr. Rick Wilson: How healthy is your life? Dr. Wilson offers a brief lecture to engage the audience on the healthy habits that can increase longevity. These habits range from proper sun protection, to exercise, and a healthier spiritual walk to reduce stress and cortisol.

Jennifer Engels, MD: Dr. Engels is a radiologist who specializes in integrative nutrition. Her passion is helping others live their healthiest, best lives. during the half day ultimate health seminar Jennifer will test participants in break out groups for metabolic syndrome.

Dr. Engels will educate Key changes that can reduce risk factors for metabolic syndrome are:
1. Exercise: At least 30 minutes of moderate exercise per day.
2. Weight loss: Losing as little as 5-10 percent of your body weight can reduce your blood pressure and risk for diabetes.
3. Smoking cessation: Smoking worsens the health consequences of metabolic syndrome and increases insulin resistance.

Complications of metabolic syndrome include diabetes, cardiovascular disease and stroke.

Tammy Kling, Bestselling Health Author, Life Coach: Kling speaks to hospitals, corporations, assisted living facilities and innovative organizations. Her energetic session inspires people to discover their gifts and life purpose. Tammy talks about the science of the brain-heart connection, and how what we think affects what we do. Her exciting seminars engage the mind, body, and soul and motivate attendees.

Disclaimer

"This publication contains the opinions and ideas of the authors and is sold with the understanding that the authors are not engaged in rendering medical, health, or any kind of personal professional services in the book. The reader should consult his or her medical, health, or other competent professional before adopting any of the suggestions in this book."

The doctor of the future will give no medicine, but will instruct his patient in the care of the human frame, in diet and in the cause and prevention of disease.

—Thomas Edison